Ethical Decision Making
in Nursing and Healthcare
Third Edition

The Symphonological Approach

Gladys L. Husted, RN, MA, PhD, is a Professor of Nursing at Duquesne University, Pittsburgh, Pennsylvania. She was awarded the title of Distinguished Professor in 1998. She received a Master's in Nursing Education from the University of Pittsburgh, where she also completed her PhD in Curriculum and Supervision. She teaches in the BSN, MSN, and PhD programs. Her main area of expertise is in bioethics, where she writes, presents workshops, consults, and does research. Her other areas of expertise are in curriculum design, instructional strategies, and theory development.

James H. Husted is an independent scholar. He is a member of the American Philosophical Association and the North American Spinoza Society. He has been a member of the high IQ societies, Mensa and Intertel. He was the Philosophy expert for Dial-An-M for Mensa, as well as the philosophy editor of *Integra*, the journal of Intertel. He guest lectures on bioethics at Duquesne University in the BSN, MSN, and PhD programs. He writes and presents workshops in the area of bioethics.

Ethical Decision Making in Nursing and Healthcare

Third Edition

The Symphonological Approach

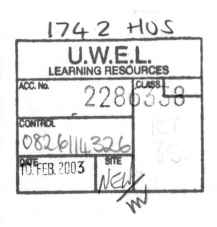

Gladys L. Husted
James H. Husted

 Springer Publishing Company

Springer Publishing Company, Inc.
536 Broadway
New York, NY 10012-3955

Acquisitions Editor: Ruth Chasek
Production Editor: Jeanne W. Libby
Cover design by Susan Hauley

02 03 04/ 5 4 3 2

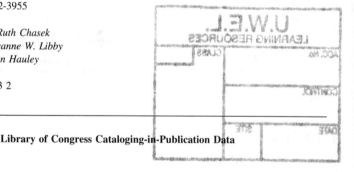

Library of Congress Cataloging-in-Publication Data

Husted, Gladys L.
   Ethical decision making in nursing and health care : the symponological approach / Gladys L. Husted, James H. Husted.—3rd ed.
      p. ; cm.
   Rev. ed. of: Ethical decision making in nursing / Gladys L. Husted, James H. Husted, 2nd ed. c1995
      Includes bibliographical references and index.
      ISBN 0-8261-1432-6
      1. Nursing ethics.   2. Nursing—Decision making.   I. Husted, James H.   II. Husted, Gladys L. Ethical decision making in nursing.   III. Title
   [DNLM: 1. Ethics, Nursing—Nurses' Instruction.   2. Decision Making—Nurses' Instruction.
   3. Models, Theoretical—Nurses' Instruction.
WY 85 H972e 2001]
RT85 .H87 2001
174'.2—dc21   2001032027

Contents

SECTION 1

The Basics of Ethical Decision Making

List of Case Study Dilemmas

List of Figures

Acknowledgments

We wish to acknowledge our gratitude to the following people:

Our **students**, who served as a crucible for refining the dominant ideas in this book.

Kirsten (Champagne) and **Gary Kalwaytis**, for sharing an adventure and the prospect of new adventures.

Tabitha and **Rich Riggio**, who gave us love, encouragement, and support.

Melanie and **Allena**, who reminded us of the seriousness of play and the appropriateness of play to seriousness.

Aubrey, for reintroducing us to Oscar Wilde.

M. Carroll Miller, a loving friend and wonderful editor.

Sharen and **David Custer**, for their enthusiasm and friendship.

Ruth Chasek, the alchemist, for her insightful and challenging editing.

Jeanne Libby, the enabler, for her patience and encouragement.

And finally to **Charlie-Charlie**, to whom this book is dedicated.

Contributors

Barbara A. Brown, RN, PhD, CCRN
Professor
Philosophy Department
Community College of Allegheny County
Pittsburgh, Pennsylvania

Marge Hardt, RN, MSN
Director of Operations and Chief Nursing Officer
West Penn Allegheny Health System
Suburban General Hospital
Pittsburgh, Pennsylvania

Kimberly C. Hopey, MS, RN
Director of Case Management
Allegheny General Hospital
West Penn Allegheny Health System
Pittsburgh, Pennsylvania

Carrie Scotto, MSN, RN
Assistant Professor
School of Nursing
Malone College
Canton, Ohio

Preface

Health care professionals today practice in a "salad bowl" society. No professional can hope to find her[1] beliefs shared by everyone in the biomedical setting. Everyone wants to act in ways he or she can believe to be ethically right. Whatever your ethical beliefs, however, you, as a professional, will be faced with the necessity of taking actions that you consider wrong.

This is not a reason for you to ignore questions of right and wrong. It is, in fact, a very important reason for you to understand your ethical beliefs. You are at a very great disadvantage if you do not understand **why** you consider one action right and another action wrong. You will be unable to interact on an equal footing with your colleagues. You will not be able to objectively and effectively defend the actions you take. You will have no objective means of moral self-defense.

PRACTICE-BASED BIOETHICS

"Symphonia" is a Greek work meaning agreement. Symphonology, then, is the study of agreements and what is necessary to the forming of agreements. For our purposes, it is the study of agreements in the health care arena between health care professionals and patients. It is a study of the ethical implications of the health care professional/patient agreement.

Symphonology is, by conscious design, a practice-based ethic appropriate to people practicing as professionals. It is a set of standards of behavior, preconditions necessary to agreement and professional interaction, requiring contextual understanding and application for ideal interactions in the health care setting.

The standards, as we have defined them, that must be applied to people in an ethical context according to their rights and responsibilities are:

- The right to **autonomy** is the right to be oneself and to value that which one desires.
- The right to **freedom** is the right to act to pursue one's own purposes without interference.
- The right to **objectivity** is the right to act on an objective view of reality and one's life without being victimized by deception or stress.
- The right to **self-assertion** is the right to use one's reason to make one's own decisions. It is the right to enjoy independent self-ownership. It is a right not to have one's agency "taken over" by another.
- The right to **beneficence** is the right not to be harmed, and to increase one's agency through stable agreements.
- The right to **fidelity** is the right to expect agreements to be kept.

Much has been written about optimum care for the patient. While optimum care for the patient is indispensable, in fact, central to professional bioethics, we have also concentrated on the welfare of the health care professional. A very high degree of personal development and emotional fulfillment for the professional is possible through bioethics. This is also central to the well-being of patients. These two aspects of the health care system can be made to "walk together." A symphonological ethic achieves this.

Although the primary concern of the book is ethical problems faced by nurses, there are some cases throughout the book dealing with other health care professions—pharmacists, physical therapists, physicians, social workers, dieticians, etc. The theory presented here is applicable to any health care profession. The only adjustment that needs to be made is consideration of the role—the education and experience of each. The theory is also applicable to any patient population, regardless of age, disease, competency, and cultural background.

OVERVIEW

We have included numerous dilemmas, many of which are similar, to give the professional practice in ethical decision making. We offer resolutions to most of the dilemmas in the book, realizing that "being there" may change the information that can be sought and, therefore, may alter the resolution. But for the purpose of practicing ethical decision making, we suggest that you deal with the context as presented.

This book covers every type of bioethical dilemma from bedwetting to euthanasia. It demonstrates the relevance of the bioethical standards to these (and by extension to all) bioethical dilemmas. It rigorously examines how the bioethical standards must be defined and understood in order to be used in ethical decision making.

This approach brings the reader into the center of the bioethical environment. The ethical decision-making process presented throughout the book should enable a person entering a nursing career to be at home in the profession more quickly.

We invite you to visit our web page at: www.nursing.duq.edu/faculty/husted/ bioethical/index.html

NOTE

1. The pronoun she/her is used to designate the health care professional. This convention is for the reader's ease of understanding and to keep understanding in context. The singular is preferred to the plural or indeterminate because professionals are individuals, and a practice-based ethic is, and ought to be, an individualistic ethic.

A Note to Educators: Using This Book as a Textbook

Carrie Scotto

The inclusion of ethical content in curricula is meant to improve quality of care by preparing professionals to act ethically and to assist them in ethical decision making. Typically, undergraduate ethics curricula include an abbreviated review of the historical progress of ethical thought. Traditional methods for making ethical decisions and the underlying philosophy for such methods are examined. The philosophical concepts addressed usually include deontology based on the work of Kant and utilitarianism with its 'basis' in the logic of mathematics. Ethical decision making based on what is socially acceptable in a given time and culture is discussed, along with the tendency to base ethical decision on emotional responses.

Following this review, principles of ethics and ethical standards are presented as absolute tenets. Rules or emotions are delineated as premises to be applied in each situation, regardless of context. The student is then encouraged to choose a philosophical framework, apply the principles, and solve particular ethical dilemmas. Many authors suggest ordered steps or formulas designed to facilitate the decision-making process.

A comparison of outcomes based on particular philosophies or frameworks often provokes philosophical discussion to determine which is most correct. These discussions are rarely conclusive and, at best, serve to demonstrate the inadequacies of most formulas and frameworks. At their worst, such discussions prompt individuals to become judgmental and suspicious of their colleagues' rightness of thought or moral attitudes. The deficiencies in traditional systems leave the instructor hard-pressed to mediate these discussions and the students less prepared to address ethical issues rationally.

An Alternative

Symphonology establishes from the start that traditional methods of ethical decision making are not adequate for situations created by modern health care. Departure from confusing and paradoxical methods allows the student freedom to consider ethical dilemmas in a realistic light.

Undergraduate students, given "permission," quickly begin to consider each situation individually rather than trying to produce an answer from a list of rules. Those with restrictive personal beliefs are better able to begin examination of a dilemma with the patient's uniqueness in mind rather than their own. Symphonology neither creates artificial boundaries around ethical dilemmas nor forces individuals to surrender their personal beliefs. Because the basis of symphonology is agreement, discussions center around understanding of commonalities and differences created by the context. Students, and all learners, are not forced to choose sides, but become concerned with what is most beneficial to their individual patient.

The practice of symphonology enables professionals to relate ethical decisions and actions directly to their nursing practice. Holland (1999) distinguished between actions that are inept and actions that are unethical. Using the example of a nurse speaking offensively to a patient, he identified this as merely inept, not unethical, behavior. With understanding of the standards of symphonology comes the knowledge that inept practice is unethical. This emphasizes for students the value of accountability and responsibility in practice and the pervasive need for ethics to one's practice.

TIPS ON THE USE OF THE TEXT FOR THE EDUCATOR

Section 1 of the text fosters the student's ability to recognize and choose ethical behavior in practice. It is useful for both undergraduate and graduate educational levels, and guides the student in developing ethical knowledge that is applicable to all situations. It establishes the foundation of ethics and ethical decision making. In presenting the material, the first five chapters provide a logical outline.

Using an example such as the following, students are guided in applying the traditional methods of bioethical decision making.

Sally is a nurse assigned to care for Mrs. Smith. A physician writes an order for a certain medication to be given to the patient. Sally is not very familiar with this medication, but knows it is used to treat conditions such as Mrs. Smith's. Sally prepares the medication as ordered and gives it to Mrs. Smith. Did Sally act ethically?

It quickly becomes apparent that no consensus can be reached. Giving more details such as, "Mrs. Smith is your grandmother and has asked for no further treatment," serves only to further muddy the waters. This sets the stage for the student to recognize the central role of context in ethics and the importance of a practice-based approach.

The following is a brief commentary on the motivating value of each chapter.

Chapter 1 begins with an amusing story about cavemen to introduce the nature of individual rights. The point of the story would be impossible to miss. It proceeds with a review of the historical development of ethical thought, including the traditional methods of ethical decision making. These will be the methods that are already part of some students' body of knowledge. The educator can help the student look at these methods critically in light of their own practice. It begins to develop the mind-set of symphonology.

Chapter 2 has excellent examples to illustrate the necessity of the interweaving of the context of the situation and the context of knowledge. Students readily begin to appreciate the skills needed to discover the context of a situation though interview, physical assessment, and an acute power of awareness/observation. A discussion of the context of knowledge is particularly meaningful in regard to responsibility and accountability in practice. The association of assessment, responsibility, and accountability with the context accentuates the connection between ethics and nursing practice.

Chapter 3 identifies what has been strangely lacking in discussions of bioethics. That is the central importance of the patient. The definitions of a patient and a professional, and the concepts of agency and the centrality of the patient are essential before moving onto an understanding of the health care professional/patient agreement. It creates a mind-set that is essential to effective and appropriate ethical decision making.

Chapter 4 clarifies the nature of the professional/patient agreement. It illustrates what is common in bioethical discussions—the importance of obligation. It relates ethical obligation, not to something outside of the nurse/patient context, but directly to the agreement they form between them. It is this that establishes their role in their relationship.

The example of the two islanders at the beginning of chapter 4 makes an engaging segue to the concept of agreement. The definition of agreement and the meaning of rights and fidelity are the subjects of the next discussion. It is helpful to revisit the islander example after a discussion of the concepts underlying the professional/patient agreement. Students with particularly strong or restrictive personal beliefs may find it difficult to maintain the centrality of the patient's desire if it conflicts with their own views. Recalling the islanders helps the student to be less resistant to discovering the inner workings of another. This done, the students are then more willing to support patients in any purpose to which they have a right.

Having gained an understanding of the nature of the professional/patient agreement, students are then ready to examine the structure of the agreement.

Chapter 5 discusses the bioethical standards as preconditions of the professional/patient agreement. It is important for the student to understand that the standards define the human obligations underlying the agreement. The bioethical standards are usually familiar to most students. It is interesting to ask the class to define the terms as they understand them and then compare their definitions with those from chapter 5. The glossary in the book is extensive and very helpful. At this time, the introduction of the Symphonological Bioethical Decision-Making Guide (Figure 5.1) helps students conceptualize the decision-making process.

Chapter 6, which for many will be the centerpiece of the text, discusses the most effective way to resolve complex and difficult cases, especially those where the proper beneficiary is not apparent. While it helps with extremely difficult cases, the chapter itself is not difficult to understand. The teacher will be able to easily help the students to grasp its central meaning.

Discussing the case studies helps clarify the meanings of the standards according to symphonology. Placing students in small groups to discuss the cases and then report their conclusions helps them to verbalize the process and concepts. After the students work through a number of cases, it is interesting to return to a prescribed formula for ethical decision making. This exercise emphasizes the lack of logic and humanity in systems that are not context-based.

Coope (1996) expressed concern that the use of case studies in teaching ethics serves to misrepresent the extent to which the choice of ethical action is controversial, and that discussion of case studies promotes the consideration of options that are immoral. The practice of symphonology eliminates these concerns because the outcome is not a matter of choosing right from wrong, but of recognizing what will most benefit the individual in question and who is the rightful beneficiary.

There are some cases in the book that are not analyzed—these are bolded. These offer further experience in ethical decision making. Because of the large number of cases that are in the text, the teacher can pick and choose which ones to have the students analyze. The cases deal with the every day ethical practice of health care professionals, as well as very complex dilemmas that are not as frequently faced.

Section 2 is useful for those who have moved beyond the basics and desire a deeper understanding of the bioethical decision-making process. These chapters provide numerous case studies appropriate for classroom discussion for all levels of learners. This section brings clarity to the understanding and practice of symphonology, and promotes growth and well-being for the patient, professional, and the profession.

Chapter 7 shows how, in all interaction, understanding is necessary, and how mutual understanding can be achieved through using the bioethical standards as lenses. The educator can use introspection to help the students reflect on the standards in relation to themselves.

Chapter 8 enables a teacher to further hone the student's abilities at ethical decision making. It does this by showing how apparent conflicts between the standards are overcome.

Chapter 9 discusses the historic understanding of human virtue and the ways in which attention to the standards as virtues can build professional competence and pride. Further, it shows the differences among ways of caring and gives the student and educator a way of preventing burn-out.

Section 3 deals with an examination of the concept of autonomy and its underlying elements. This section is particularly appropriate for the educator, for the registered nurse returning to school, for those students receiving advanced degrees, and for the scholar interested in bioethics. This section deals with the philosophy of human nature and human action and interaction, as well as the philosophical underpinnings of symphonology. The Symphonological Bioethical Decision-Making Advanced Guide (Figure 10.1) illustrates the interrelationships of the concepts in the decision-making process with the added addition of the elements of autonomy. Many case studies are offered that can be used for classroom discussion. The educator should be aware of the advanced nature of the resolutions resolved through the elements of human autonomy, but masters' and doctoral students are quick to be able to use the elements.

Chapter 10 shows the supreme importance of human autonomy. The chapter demonstrates how individual autonomy is framed through the elements of desire, reason, life, purpose, and agency. The importance of considering a person's autonomy when making decisions is further explicated. In doing this, the chapter discusses:

1. The relationship between human desire and ethical concerns.
2. The importance of reasoning (critical thinking) to practice-based decision making.
3. How different views of life impact on ethical decision making.
4. How human purposes relate to ethical concerns—showing their identity.
5. How the exercise and the requirements of agency are central ethical concerns of the health care system.

Chapter 11 delineates the theoretical and philosophical underpinnings of symphonology. For most students, it will not be of central importance, unless the student is taking a doctoral-level course in bioethics, a theory course, or has a specific interest in bioethics. It is, of course, a must for the educator. While it is not necessary to the understanding of symphonological bioethical decision making, it is well-worth the effort to, at least, review.

Section 4 looks at the relationship of symphonology to agreements other than the clinician/patient agreement.

Chapter 12 discusses the educator/student/patient agreement.

Chapter 13 discusses the administrator/professional/patient agreement.

Chapter 14 discusses the researcher/subject agreement.

Chapter 15 discusses the health care professional/patient agreement and advance directives.

The reader should note that in each of these topics, the primary beneficiary must always be included in the agreement—in every case, this is the patient or subject in the case of research. No matter what role a professional assumes—educator, administrator, researcher, or consultant—her primary concern must be the patient and the patient's welfare.

Section 5 provides analysis and explanation of marked case studies throughout the text. This is a significant strength of the book and is very helpful in the teaching/learning process.

REFERENCES

Coope, C. (1996). Does teaching by case study mislead us about morality? *Journal of Medical Ethics, 22*, 46–52.

Holland, S. (1999). Teaching nursing ethics by cases: A personal perspective. *Nursing Ethics, 6*, 434–436.

The Basics of Ethical Decision Making

CHAPTER 1

A Critical History of Ethics

One day, many thousands of years ago, two cavemen passed each other on a forest pathway. One caveman struck the other with a club and knocked him down. There was nothing unusual about this. It had happened between cavemen many times before and it has happened between cavemen many times since. (It happens all the time.) But this day, something world-historic happened. The victim, holding his bloodied head, looked up and asked the fateful question, "Why did you do that?" This was history's first demand for an ethical justification.

Unfortunately for the children of cavemen, on that day the aggressor caveman did not bother to reply. At that time, cavemen did not spend much time analyzing ethical dilemmas.

Thousands of years later, the same event occurred on an even more remarkable day, but with one noticeable difference: The aggressor replied to his victim's query with the remark: "I harm you so that you will have no power to harm me. It is terribly unfortunate that you and I cannot leave each other alone, each free to do what he wants to do. Someday, we ought to give some thought to this."

More time passed. During this passage of time, the human race began to form the idea of individual rights—the right to be left alone. It is an idea with a very rocky history and one that is far from completely formed. But it is a reality. It does motivate and control much human interaction. One can observe this reality in operation constantly and everywhere. It is the irreplaceable reality determining humanity's ethical existence.

Rights* is produced by an implicit agreement among rational beings, which they make and hold by virtue of their rationality—their ability to think. It is an agreement that they will not force one another to take action and that they will not steal the values that an individual's actions have produced. This agreement establishes the practice of acting together only on the basis of the voluntary consent of everyone involved—a consent that is obtained without deception.

Rights is: The product of an implicit agreement among rational beings, made and held by virtue of their rationality, not to obtain actions or the product of actions from each other except through voluntary consent, objectively gained.

Rights pertains to an individual's freedom of action. An individual has a right to make free choices among alternatives based on his or her desires, purposes, and values.

In a state of solitude, a person has a 'right' to do whatever he or she is capable of doing. An individual has this right in the sense that no one else is relevantly involved and there is no possibility of violating the rights of others.

The benefit of this agreement is so great and so obvious, the detriment of not having this agreement is so manifestly ruinous, that the agreement literally "goes without saying." It is, in various ways, the basis of all benevolence and cooperation among people.

As cavemen became more and more rational, they began to form this agreement among themselves. It was formed naturally and spontaneously, simply as a matter of course. It is an agreement to forego aggression in favor of discussion and agreement.

As reason began to enlighten their lives, cavemen realized that aggression is dysfunctional and that nothing produces human progress and well-being more perfectly than free and informed cooperation. The practice of recognizing rights spread. The process still continues. It is often inconvenient but always alluring. In the long run, nothing else makes sense. When this agreement is put aside, there is nothing whatsoever to protect people against each other's brutal irrationality or to assure good faith and justice in their interactions.

The recognition of rights is an essential element of the ethical interaction between nurse and patient. It is an original and implicit agreement that shapes every future agreement.

THE PHILOSOPHY OF ETHICS

Ethics, like every science, arose from the necessity of making decisions in the face of adversity.

---

*As the reader proceeds through the text, the necessity of regarding "rights" as a singular concept, denoting a single, noncomplex agreement, will become obvious.

Every field of study has a purpose. Human beings needed to navigate the seas; someone created astronomy. Curious about living things, someone created biology. Someone created mathematics for the purpose of computation. Someone created medicine from a desire to heal. Every science and every art arises from imagination and reason. These are inspired by need or curiosity. This is as true of ethics—the science of living well—as it is for all other fields of study.

Socrates, the founder of ethics in the Western world, was not the first person ever to think about very basic human problems. He was, however, probably the first to think about them deeply and rigorously. He proposed a systematic examination of human experience and human life as the way to discover solutions. He discovered the necessity of doubt. This began that part of philosophy that is known as ethics. Ethics examines the ways men and women can exercise their power in order to bring about human benefit—the ways in which we can act in order to bring about the conditions of happiness.

Sciences deal with alternatives. For ethics, the central alternative is between the beneficial (the "good") and the harmful (the "evil"). In an ethical context, that which increases human welfare is the good and that which is contrary to human welfare is the evil. In an ethical sense, a failed life is one which, at the end, one looks back on with disappointment. A successful life is a life that one experiences as having been worth living.

The demands of successful living are the natural principles of ethics. For instance, an individual requires the virtue of courage—a willingness to meet the demands that a human life makes—in order to live successfully (Plato in Jowett, 1937). This makes courage one of the natural principles of ethics.

In a derivative way, ethics also involves a study of the interactions between ethical agents. This study is made in terms of right and wrong. It deals with the ethical conditions of interaction. These are the conditions under which one agent has, or has not, the right to expect to benefit from the action of another.

Ethics looks to the human condition and its relation to what is appropriate to human interactions. It is concerned with the nature of the goals that agents ought to pursue together. It discovers the ways these goals ought to be pursued. Ethics examines the decisions and choices agents ought to make in regard to their interactions.

In relation to these decisions and choices, the right is that which is based on objective agreement. The wrong is that which involves deception or coercion.

In the nature of interaction, it is possible for intentions to be right and consequences to be bad. Unknown conditions and unforeseeable events are never irrelevant to the consequences of action or interaction. It is also possible, although extremely unusual, for intentions to be wrong and consequences to be good. Deception and coercion, by their natures, do not serve human action and life.

Ethics examines the processes of decision making and the ways in which agents reach, or fail to reach, their goals.

For all of these reasons, ethics has traditionally been called "the practical science." The ability to engage in processes of ethical analysis is known as "practical reason." "[Since] ethics is fundamentally a practical discipline [it is] concerned with what we should do and how we should live . . . " (Churchill, 1989, p. 28).

THE BIRTH OF BIOETHICS

In order for a new science to be discovered, certain conditions are necessary:

1. The science must yield very abstract and general knowledge. There can be no science of crab apple trees. The discovery of how the speed of hair growth can be predicted would not constitute a science. These subjects are too narrow. Science is concerned with very broad areas of human interest.
2. There must be a purpose for the discovery. If it fills no need, it cannot be a science. There is no scientific way to harness flying horses. There is no possibility of anyone needing to harness a flying horse.
3. It must be possible to make the discovery. There must be something out in the world to be discovered. There can be no science of time travel. So far, at least, no one has made progress toward time travel.
4. The discoverer must love the pursuit of knowledge and have a tireless curiosity concerning the subject matter.

A certain Athenian possessed these qualities in abundance. He is, perhaps, the most famous philosopher of the Western world. The adventure of his discovery has been immortalized in the *Dialogues of Plato*. The adventure began in ancient Greece about 450 B.C.

Inspired by the belief that "The unexamined life is not worth living," Socrates was the first philosopher to systematically turn his attention to the affairs of human life. Socrates, the son of a stone mason and a midwife, saw himself as following his mother's profession, with this difference:

Where his mother assisted at the birth of children, he assisted at the birth of ideas. This he did through a method that he called dialectic. The method involved disciplined conversation. Socrates would begin by posing a question. When a member of his audience offered an answer, he would question the answer. Through this method (which has come to be known as the maieutic method—the method of midwifery), Socrates led his audience to make ethical inductions. That is to say, by reflecting on concrete facts, they were led to wide-ranging ethical understanding.

Socrates was convinced that no virtue and no ethical action is possible without knowledge. He also believed that no ethical knowledge is possible without an understanding of the meaning of ethical terms. To have a knowledge of virtuous action one must first know what virtue is. To gain an understanding of actions as just or unjust one must understand the essential nature of justice. To know the requirements of happiness one must first know the defining properties of happiness (Plato in Jowett, 1937).

These conversations often led the people of Athens into areas where they had no desire to go. Their ethical beliefs consisted entirely of social customs and conventions. To engage them in practical reasoning, Socrates had to call their beliefs into question. To have one's beliefs called into question is a painful experience. To call one's own beliefs into question is a very unpopular activity. But no practical reasoning is possible without this activity and this experience.

As is well known, Socrates' curiosity cost him his life. He was executed by the state for teaching heresy and "corrupting the youth of Athens." Then, as now, many people would rather kill, or die, before engaging in practical reasoning (Vlastos, 1991).

BIOETHICS

Bioethics—ethics as it relates to the health care professions—came into existence as an independent discipline about 1970: " . . . the vocabulary of the moral—of right and wrong—has been added to the vocabulary of scientific medicine—of fact and content" (Cassell, 1984, p. 35).

The development of bioethics has been more like Socrates' method of dialectic than anything that has occurred in ethics in 2,500 years. Many factors—cultural, legal, philosophic—have set the direction of this development.

The fundamental background of bioethics, which forms its essential nature, is:

- The nature and needs of humans as living, thinking beings.
- The purpose and function of the health care system in a human society.
- An increased cultural awareness of human beings' essential moral status.

All this forms the nature of the biomedical context. The needs and conditions of people who enter this context do not allow for the nonobjective, the purposeless, or the arbitrary. The interpersonal relationships of health care professionals and patients give added dimension to this context. The values, which the biomedical sciences offer those who can profit from them, are complex and vitally important.

At the same time, the threat to a patient's values is very real. The relationship between the health care professional and patient is extraordinarily intimate. At the present time, it may well be deteriorating.

Health care professionals possess an undesirable degree of power over patients. They may be tempted to take actions that can be justified only through rationalization. They are sometimes motivated to take irrelevant, ritualistic actions. They often have little concern for the ethical meaning of their actions. They may see little need for ethical doubt or analysis. Their ethical concerns may be misguided. Their patients are vulnerable.

Biomedicine, at its best, is reality oriented, well reasoned, and centered on the individual. It is not desirable and not necessary that bioethics should differ from the medical professions in this regard. To protect these elements of professional practice, it is necessary—and desirable—that bioethics should be practice-based.

ETHICS AS PRACTICE-BASED

Bioethics as a practice-based ethic has the purpose of enhancing the benefits available through the health care system. The decision-making principles presented here are the commonly accepted ideals of the biomedical professions. They are the natural principles of all interaction. They not only serve as guides to bioethical decision making and action but they are, themselves, ethical decisions.

They are decisions reached by thousands of health care professionals through decades of experience—the experience of that which succeeds and is right and the experience of that which fails and is wrong. These decision-making principles are:

- Every patient has a right to be treated according to his* unique character-structure.
- Every patient has a right to decide and act on his own values to fulfill his own life plans.
- Every patient has a right to expect complete and objective information and the emotional support necessary to act effectively on that information.
- Every patient has the right, alone or through a health care professional, to the control of his time and effort.
- Every patient has a right to expect whatever benefit is possible in the health care setting, and to expect no avoidable harm.
- Every patient has a right to expect that agreements established with health care professionals will be kept.

The bioethical principles are generally accepted. They are, at least, given lip service. They are tools of justification, internal to professional practice. They are not always consistently applied. When they are not applied, they produce first comedy, then tragedy, in the health care setting. The unique character-structure of individual patients is often ignored. Patients may be treated as interchangeable. No justification is ever given for this treatment. Such a justification would be comical. The dehumanizing effects of this on patients and health care professionals

---

*Note: For clarity's sake the masculine pronoun will be used for the patient. As mentioned in the Preface, the female pronoun will be used for the health professional.

are tragic. Health care professionals often compel or deceive patients into acting against the patient's rights and values. To assume that this is proper is comical. The erosion of individual rights that it causes is tragic. Sometimes, it is assumed that a patient has no right to awareness of what is happening in and to his life. Imagine someone trying to justify this with a straight face. Try to envision the effect this has on human life. What ethical or logical processes could produce this idea? It is a tragedy. Do patients have no right to expect benefits in the health care setting or to be protected from harm? No one believes this, at least not explicitly.

These ideas are all comical. But sometimes the comical comes to appear reasonable. Between persons, especially persons in the health care system, an agreement can be made that they will interact with the maximum possible benevolence. This agreement can be kept. Since it can be made and kept, when it is not, it is tragic.

THE HEALTH CARE PROFESSIONAL/PATIENT AGREEMENT

In a primary sense, ethical actions are the actions an individual takes in the pursuit of his or her vital and fundamental goals. These are the actions that inspired the study of ethics. Actions involving the rights of others are also ethical actions. The actions that a health care professional takes in her role as professional always have an ethical aspect. They are always concerned with vital and fundamental goals. In her role as professional, she acts as agent for her patient. This is a complex ethical relationship.

Every human relationship arises from an explicit or implicit agreement. The relationship that arises between a professional and patient is one instance of this. The principles by which a professional makes a decision ought to be derived from the actual dynamics of this agreement. The dynamics of the agreement are formed by the values a patient seeks to attain, maintain, or regain in the relationship. On the professional's part, they are the values that she agrees to help her patient realize.

A patient, in becoming a patient, has a specific purpose. A professional, in becoming a professional, takes on a specific role. Their purposes interface. They interface by design. The purpose of a patient (regaining, attaining, or maintaining the power of agency) determines the role of a professional.

A professional, in becoming a professional, becomes the agent of her patient. A professional does for her patient what the patient would do for himself had he not lost his power of agency. She assists him in achieving the ability to take independent actions.

The interrelationship between them is formed by the nature of a professional (one who acts for a patient) and the nature of a patient (one who lacks the power to act for himself). In the interaction of professional and patient, their roles form an implicit agreement between them. They agree, in effect, that, since the patient is a patient, the professional will be a professional. The entire area of a professional's ethical action lies within these parameters.

THE STRUCTURE OF AN ETHICAL CODE ILLUSTRATED

In the natural course of life, a person will, of necessity, adopt an ethical code. The code adopted may be Plato's (the pursuit of an unknowable Final Good), Immanuel Kant's deontology (action according to the demands of duty), John Stuart Mill's utilitarianism ("the greatest good of the greatest number" as the highest ethical goal), Uncle Dick's, Aunt Jane's, or the voice of inner urges. But a person cannot evade the need to find some way of ordering his or her life.

The function of an ethical code is similar in some ways to the function of a travel agent. In order to examine that which is unfamiliar, the inner structure of an ethical code, we can have recourse to that which is more familiar, the itinerary of a vacation.

A vacation involves: The time of departure—precisely when one will leave to go on vacation; the time of arrival—when one can expect to reach one's destination; the time when one will leave the vacation spot to return home; the location where one is going to spend one's vacation and the attractions and facilities that are found there; where one will stay—the accommodations one can expect and how accessible everything will be; the means of transportation to and from one's vacation spot; the cost of one's vacation; and the luggage one should take.

Would any sensible person put his entire vacation into the hands of a travel agent? Would he let the agent decide when to leave; where to go; how long to stay; when to return home; where to stay; how to get there; and the cost of the vacation?

The choice among vacation spots would be made according to the travel agent's evaluations. The traveler's desires would play no part in the planning of the vacation.

No sensible person would agree to this arrangement. Yet, incredibly, many otherwise thinking people will make this arrangement with an ethical theory that they have chosen, or have had chosen for them, at random. In terms of this ethical theory, they plan the purpose and course of their entire life. The ethical theory and their responsibilities to the role they take on in their lives may go in entirely different directions.

In our culture, at this time, two broad theories of ethics are dominant.

Deontology

Deontology makes right and wrong the central ethical concepts. Ethical action consists in doing one's duty. To do one's duty is right. To shirk one's duty is wrong. The ethical agent has a duty to do what is right and to refrain from doing what is wrong. Beyond this, nothing is ethically relevant. The results of an action may be desired or deplored, but they have no ethical relevance.

The notion of duty as central to ethics arose with the Stoic philosophers about 300 B.C., but its most powerful impetus was given by the German philosopher Immanuel Kant (1724–1804).

The concept of duty is unrelated to our everyday concerns. Kant's duty-ethic was a reaction to the social-subjectivism of David Hume (1711–1776) ("X is right" means society approves X; "X is wrong" means society disapproves of X). In turn, all Kantian-type ethics were attacked by the English philosopher G. E. Moore (1873–1958). Moore described the attempt to get an "ought" (a duty) from an "is" (a fact relevant to human existence) as a fallacious mode of thinking. He named this the naturalistic fallacy (Schilpp, 1968).

Ought and right are both defined by a duty ethic in terms of duty. This makes a duty ethic viciously circular. The right is that which one ought to do (has a duty to do) because one ought to do that which is right (that which one has a duty to do). This is done for no reason other than that the right is that which one ought to do (Hospers, 1967).

No deontologist has ever found the reason for duty in the demands of human life. The Stoics located it in a Platonist "World-Soul." The duties of people, the revolutions of the sun, the wetness of water are all part of the same thing—the laws that govern nature.

There is a logical drawback to this. It proves that which is doubtful (that people have duties) in terms of that which is even more doubtful (the existence of Plato's "World-Soul"). It is like proving that Jane will be in town at noon (a doubtful possibility) by declaring that Martians will "beam" her to town at noon (a much more doubtful possibility).

Kant held that the concept of duty is an innate idea. One is born knowing that he must do his duty and what his duty is (Kant, 1785/1964). This notion is also highly doubtful. In order to know the demands of duty laid upon him, a newborn would need to know of the relationships existing between himself and the world. In order to know this, he would need to know of the nature of the world. He would need to know this before knowing that there is a world. This is impossible.

Historically, notions of duty and the right have been in flux. Every neighboring culture and every succeeding age has its own view of the right. Every era and culture is entirely convinced that its view of the right is part of the makeup of the natural world.

Deontology demands that right actions be taken without regard to consequences. A nurse cannot justify taking an action without concern for the effects they will produce. She should always be able to justify her actions in terms of their (foreseeable) consequences.

> Deontological ethics maintains that, if one acts from a genuine sense of moral duty,
> then one's action is morally approvable irrespective of its actual conse-
> quences. . . . [But] the deliberate ignoring of foreseeable consequences of one's
> actions is an abandonment of the primary function of Practical Reasoning. . . . [This
> is in opposition to the] virtuous capacity of the good person to look forward to the
> most likely results of a given decision or voluntary act (Bourke, 1983, p. 10).

Could a nurse justify causing harm to a patient by saying "I was doing my
duty?" This would not suffice legally. It surely does not suffice ethically—not if
ethically is understood in any practical or rational sense.

If the purpose of an ethical system is to serve human life—or the efficient
functioning of a profession—then deontology is not an ethical system. It is the
absence of an ethical system. Consider this: The original deontologists preached
the rightness of duty in action. They saw that a certain state of mind must,
necessarily, follow these actions. The permanent possession of this state of mind
was the purpose of deontology.

The Stoics called this state of mind apatheia, which means a state of apathy
produced by living in the straightjacket of deontology. A modern name for this
state is burn-out. Apathy demands indifference to pain or pleasure, health or
illness, happiness or misery. The father of modern deontology, Immanuel Kant,
sings the praises of apathy in the preface to *Groundwork for the Metaphysics of
Morals* in a section entitled, "Virtue Necessarily Presupposes Apathy (Considered
as Strength)" (1964).

Indifference is an undesirable quality in a nurse. It is the opposite of what a
nurse's state of mind ought to be. But one cannot, consistently, practice deontology
without it. The practice of a duty ethic has never benefitted patients or nursing—and
certainly not individual nurses.

Nevertheless, many ethicists regard duty and morality as equivalent terms.
They claim that ethics and deontology are identical. If this is true, then the only
task of ethics is to list a person's duties, and every ethical action is simply an act
of obedience. "The idea that we are following rules when we act morally is a
tired hangover from the days when the lives of people were controlled by religious
and secular absolute rulers who accorded no respect or autonomy [independence]
to ordinary people" (van Hooft, 1990, p. 211).

Nurses cannot escape taking the role of ethical agent. One option open to a
nurse is to answer the demands of her innate and prerational sense of duty. To
do this, she must be aware of having an innate and prerational sense of duty. No
one can ever be certain that an innate idea is true. Worse than this, no one can
ever be certain that any idea is innate. The only way she could be certain that an
idea is innate is to contrast it with an idea that she learns from her experience.
An innate idea is an idea that one has not learned from experience. Which means
that, an innate idea is an idea that one has no reason to believe (Benner, 1984).

Dilemma 1-1   Zelda believes that she has a duty to give cardiac patients detailed information on the pathology involved in their condition. Mr. Wu and Mr. Goldfarb are two cardiac patients assigned to her. Mr. Wu is very much interested in having this information. But, to Mr. Goldfarb, it is terrifying. He is greatly depressed by her recitation.

Had Zelda respected the uniqueness of Mr. Goldfarb, she would have given him only that information that would have been of benefit to him and that would have caused him no unnecessary stress. She would have been motivated by beneficence rather than by her sense of duty. This would have necessitated a betrayal of the best interests of deontology. It is not difficult to see that her fidelity to duty was a betrayal of the best interests of Mr. Goldfarb. But, insofar as duty is Zelda's ethical standard, there is no significant ethical difference between Zelda's relationship to Mr. Goldfarb and her relationship to Mr. Wu.

Deontology is entirely concerned with an agent's actions. It is unconcerned with consequences. It is also indifferent to the agent's intentions, except his intention to do his duty. In principle, deontology demands indifference to individual autonomy. The recognition of autonomy would require that a nurse make choices appropriate to the uniqueness of her patient. Yet, in deontology, the demands of duty are imperative—they do not allow for choices to be made on the part of a nurse. Autonomous differences among patients call for a nurse to analyze each situation. A deontologist who analyzed contextual differences and made choices based on her analysis would have, perhaps unknowingly, abandoned deontology.

Utilitarianism

The central ethical concepts of utilitarianism are good and evil. Utilitarianism finds its basis in the doctrine of psychological hedonism. Psychological hedonism is a form of determinism. Hedonism is the doctrine that ethical agents are, and ought to be, motivated solely by pleasure or pain. David Hume's (1955) famous aphorism, "Reason is, and rightly ought to be, the slave of the passions [emotions]," would serve as a motto for hedonism.

Utilitarianism was first formulated in terms of psychological hedonism, which means that determinism was the first inspiration of utilitarianism.

Determinism is the doctrine that every human action is a response to a prior event. This prior event originates outside of the person who is (apparently) acting. The determinist holds that deciding and choosing are illusions. Determinists have described the feeling of being able to control one's thoughts and actions as a kind of dream. Psychological hedonism is a form of determinism. It is the doctrine that every action of an agent is, of necessity, a response to the experience or the expectation of pleasure or pain. It holds that one acts only to seek pleasure and to avoid pain and holds that one cannot act otherwise. It describes this tendency as being inborn (Hospers, 1972).

Utilitarians claimed that people cannot escape holding pleasure to be the good. Their next step was to argue for the necessity of:

> ... the principle which approves or disapproves of every action whatsoever according to the tendency which it appears to have to augment or diminish the happiness of the party whose interest is in question. ... (Bentham, 1879/1962)

Then, they went on to argue, in effect, that the good of two persons is a greater good than the good of one. The greatest possible good, then, would be the good of everyone, or, the good of the greatest possible number. This good, they declared, ought to be the goal of every ethical agent.

Early opponents were quick to point out flaws in this reasoning. Thomas Carlyle (1795–1881) called utilitarianism a "pig philosophy." He noted that, in every conceivable way, a symphony by Beethoven was a greater good than the victory of a pig wrestler. In fact, Beethoven's creativity, from every point of view, seems a greater good than the victories of a large number of pig wrestlers (Trail, 1896).

In response to this, utilitarians amended their principle to read, "The greatest (or highest) good of the greatest number." This reasoning ignores several relevant facts:

1. Let us grant that a person, through psychological necessity, holds his own pleasure to be an end in itself. This fact, in itself, gives him no reason, logical or otherwise, to concern himself with the good of others. A person might hold his good to be of value to him not because it is a good, but because it is **his** good. There is no logical flaw in this attitude, and any claim that it is ethically flawed begs the question.

There is no rational reason for an agent to believe that his good is freely interchangeable with the good of other agents. His own good might be uniquely valued by him. He might hold that, if it is computed along with the good of another, it loses its ethical relevance.

Let us imagine someone for whom this is not the case.

Joe is very excited about going to a rock concert. Sally tells him that she is also going. Now, Joe is no longer excited. If Sally is going, it does not matter to Joe whether he goes as long as someone goes. Joe regards values as interchangeable.

Psychologically, this does not make sense. But it is utilitarianism's view of human nature.

2. It is difficult to see how a nurse could justify actions by reference to "the greatest good for the greatest number." Her primary responsibility is to her individual patient. Her patient, in turn, has a right to choose his own goals and the consequences he seeks. He has a right to choose highly individualistic goals based solely on his own desires.

> Utilitarianism not only directs us to consider the results of an action when making moral judgments but also holds that we should look only to results. Considerations of an agent's intentions, feelings, or convictions are seen as irrelevant to the question "What is the right thing to do?" (Arras & Hunt cited in Arras & Rhoden, 1989, p. 8)

A nurse in pursuit of "the greatest good of the greatest number" would have no time to attend to her individual patients. Nor would they have any right to expect individualized nursing treatment from her. Being a nurse would not allow her to take ethical action. It would be a wall between her and the possibility of ethical action.

3. Utilitarianism collapses into deontology (Veatch, 1985). This has finally been recognized even by utilitarians. To avoid this flaw, a distinction is drawn between "rule" and "act" utilitarianism. Rule utilitarians claim that an agent has a duty to obey certain rules. These are the rules best adapted to bring about the greatest good for the greatest number. Act utilitarians declare that the value of an action is determined by its goal. This simply means that an agent has a duty to aim for a specific goal. He has a duty to act to bring about the greatest good for the greatest number. Utilitarians cannot escape deontology.

4. Utilitarianism is also an ethical theory peculiar in this: Justice is the most highly honored interpersonal virtue of our society. It is the goal of our entire legal system. Ironically, utilitarianism is a prescription for injustice.

> One such limitation [of utilitarianism as an ethical theory] is the violation of personal autonomy . . . its inherent potential for discrimination, the possibility that what is perceived as "good" for the majority may be bad for the minority (Franklin, 1988, p. 35).

In fact, it is somewhat worse than that:

> Utilitarianism . . . has fallen into bad odor, and particularly when it comes to a defense of individual rights and personal liberties . . . suppose . . . the general welfare of the community, or the greatest happiness of the greatest number, might conceivably be furthered or increased by the sacrifice of the liberty, or the well-being, or even the life of a single individual. . . . [Would not this sacrifice be] . . . the moral consequence of anyone's adhering strictly to Utilitarian principles (Veatch, 1985, pp. 30–31).

Nevertheless, utilitarianism is today's dominant ethical trend. Many nursing-ethics textbooks recommend it as a tool for ethical decision making. It is an alternative theory that a nurse might want to consider. But:

> Utilitarianism requires an agent to do that action which brings about the greatest balance of good over evil in the universe as a whole . . . to maximize the good of all humans . . . to consider all of the available alternatives and perform that act which will maximize the good of all affected parties. (McConnell, 1982, p. 14)

This is utilitarianism. Does it not seem unreasonable to expect a nurse to know:

- What action will bring about "the greatest balance of good over evil in the universe as a whole"?
- What the nature of "the greatest balance of good over evil in the universe as a whole" would be?
- How one might "maximize the good of all humans"?
- The precise number of "all of the available alternatives"?
- Precisely that "act which will maximize the good of all affected parties"?

Suppose that, by some miracle, the nurse could know all this. Even then, how could utilitarianism be justified in a health care system that places a high value on the individual's rights and autonomy?

The utilitarian's ethical advice consists in emotionally charged, high-flying, and empty phrases urging on to the pursuit of the impossible. It is an impractical approach to the practical science. If an agent accepts the necessity of doing the impossible, she will become a fanatic or she will do nothing.

Dilemma 1-2 Harry is in the hospital. He is dying. Harry's family is unaware of the fact that he is dying. He does not want his family to know. Harry's son has been discharged from the army and is returning home. The family intends to surprise Harry with his son's return when he arrives home. What should be done?

A utilitarian would say that Harry's family should be advised of his prognosis, even against his wishes. They need to know this in order to decide what they desire to do. They are the greater number. Yet the standard of self-assertion would inspire Harry's nurse to keep her agreement with her patient. His right to control his time and effort would compel her to reveal the fact of his son's return and let Harry decide what he desires to do.

But, for a utilitarian, any claim of "the greatest good for the greatest number" is a sufficient reason to divulge anything or to conceal anything. Obviously, this is incompatible with the nurse/patient agreement as that agreement is usually understood.

MUSINGS

Ethics is not a mere adornment to human life. It is the science of successful human life. This has been obvious since humanity first began to consider ethical ideas. It has always been obvious in itself, but not always obvious to the people who might benefit from ethical understanding. For various reasons, ethics, while it is given much lip service, is seldom taken seriously.

The alternatives to clearly and objectively defined ethical ideas lead, not toward but away from successful living. Ethical ideas appropriate to the health science professions can, as we shall see, enormously enhance professional practice and a professional's life.

REFERENCES

Arras, J., & Rhoden, N. (Eds.). (1989). *Ethical issues in modern medicine* (3rd ed.). Mountain View, CA: Mayfield Publishing.

Benner, P. (1984). *From novice to expert*. Menlo Park, CA: Addison-Wesley.

Bentham, J. (1962). *The works of Jeremy Bentham*. (J. Bowring, Ed.). New York: Russell & Russell. (Original work published 1879)

Bourke, V. (1983, May). *The teleological and deontological dichotomy*. Paper presented at Duquesne University's First Annual Ethics Conference, Pittsburgh, PA.

Cassell, E. J. (1984). Life as a work of art. *Hastings Center Report, 14*(4), 35–37.

Churchill, L. R. (1989). Reviving a distinctive medical ethic. *Hastings Center Report, 19*(3), 28–30.

Franklin, C. (1988). Commentary on case study. *Hastings Center Report, 18*(6), 35–36.

Hospers, J. (1967). *An introduction to philosophical analysis* (2nd ed.). Englewood Cliffs, NJ: Prentice-Hall.

Hospers, J. (1972). *Human conduct*. New York: Harcourt Brace Jovanovich.

Hume, D. (1955). *Enquiry concerning the principles of morals*. New York: Handel. (Original work published in London, 1748)

Jowett, M. A. (Trans.). (1937). *The dialogues of Plato*. New York: Random House.

Kant, I. (1964). *Groundwork for the metaphysics of morals* (J. H. Paton, Trans.). New York: Harper & Row. (Original work published 1785)

McConnell, T. C. (1982). *Moral issues in health care*. Monterey, CA: Wadsworth Health Science Division.

Schilpp, P. A. (Ed.). (1968). *The philosophy of G. E. Moore* (Vol. B). LaSalle, IL: Open Court.

Trail, H. N. (Ed.). (1896). *The centenary edition of Carlyle's work*. New York: Oxford.

van Hooft, S. (1990). Moral education for nursing decisions. *Journal of Advanced Nursing, 15*, 210–215.

Veatch, H. B. (1985). *Human rights: Fact or fancy?* Baton Rouge, LA: Louisiana State University Press.

Vlastos, G. (1991). *Socrates, ironist and moral philosopher*. New York: Cornell Press.

CHAPTER 2

The Nature of the Ethical Context

I magine this scene:
　　Your name is Alice.
　　You are the Alice in Lewis Carroll's Wonderland.
You work in a kitchen in Wonderland.
The ethic of the kitchen is harsh, badly proportioned, and unjust.
If you drop an egg and fail to report having dropped it, an unhappy child will go to bed hungry.
So, if you drop an egg and want to prevent a child's unhappiness, you ought to report that you have dropped it.
Last time one of the kitchen workers dropped an egg and reported it, the Queen of Hearts had her beheaded.
You are in a perilous situation—one where you ought to think very carefully before reporting the loss of an egg.
Very seldom is the context of an ethical situation as clear-cut as this. But, in a very basic way, the context is relevant to every ethical decision and action.
If you decide to report the fact that you dropped the egg, this will be an ethical decision. It may make a child very happy. It may also be the last ethical decision you will ever make.
Imagine the character of a child who would be happy about your decision if he or she knew the particulars (the context) of it.
If you decide not to report the fact that you dropped the egg, this will also be an ethical decision. Unlike many ethical decisions, it would be a contextual, well proportioned, and rational decision.

THE NATURE OF A CONTEXT

A context is the interweaving of the relevant facts of a situation—the facts it is necessary to act upon to bring about a desired result—and the knowledge one has of how to deal most effectively with these facts.
A context consists of two distinct but dynamically interrelated elements.
The context of the situation is the aspects of a situation that are helpful to understanding the situation and to acting effectively in it. The variables that a health care professional finds within her patient's situation form the context of the situation. Every time a health care professional takes on the care of a patient, this action places her in a context. Factors, such as the patient's history and physical findings, the physician's diagnosis, the patient's family situation, laboratory results, the emotional state of the patient, and the age and sex of the patient form the context of a health care situation.

The inter-relations among the patient's medical condition, his circumstances, plans for the future, his motivations, and the resources of his character are aspects of an ethical situation. How these relate to his fundamental desires, his purposes, and his need to regain a state of agency[1] are part of the context of the situation. Decisions and actions concerning his vital and fundamental goals relate or fail to relate to the ethical situation.

The context of knowledge is an agent's preexisting knowledge[2] and present awareness of the relevant aspects of the situation. These are the aspects that are necessary to understanding the situation and to acting effectively in it. The forming of a context of knowledge is the purpose of an assessment. A health care professional needs to become aware of the relevant aspects of her patient's situation. She needs this knowledge so that she can give care based on a specific patient's actual situation. She uses her knowledge to group and prioritize the relevant aspects (the context) of the situation. In order to formulate an individualized plan of care a nurse calls on her context of knowledge in order to achieve objective awareness of the situation.

This is the context of the nurse's technical knowledge. The context of her ethical knowledge includes the knowledge of her patient as an ethical being, his relationship to the ethical—the vital and fundamental—aspects of his life. Her awareness of his ethical relation to himself—the physical, cognitive, emotional, and spiritual resources he can bring to bear to achieve benefit and avoid harm—forms her contextual ethical knowledge.

To have objective awareness is to bring what is already known to bear on the problem of what needs to be known and what can be known of the situation in order to determine the possibilities for gain and loss in regard to a patient's human values. Solving a problem requires that the elements of the problem be understandable. If they are not understandable, then some way must be found to make them understandable. Facts need to be identified, collected, and sorted in order to be put into a meaningful pattern (Polanyi, 1958).

Dilemma 2-1   Yvonne, a nurse, is treating Steve, a recovering stroke patient. Steve is having difficulty feeding himself. If Yvonne takes time to feed him, this might certainly be interpreted as an act of beneficence. It also might be interpreted as an act of interfering with his freedom. In order to exercise his freedom in the future, Steve must learn to feed himself.

On the other hand, if Yvonne tells Steve that she will not help him, that he is going to have to feed himself, this might be interpreted as a failure of beneficence. It might also be interpreted as an act by which Yvonne supports Steve's freedom of action.

The ethical context produces the ethical dilemma, and it is by reference to the context that an ethical dilemma is resolved. Yvonne's context (and every context) has three aspects:

- The situation that Yvonne faces, which calls for her to take some ethical action.
- Yvonne's awareness of the nature of the situation.
- Yvonne's preexisting beliefs concerning the standards or goals of ethical action.

Yvonne's situation calls for an ethical response. None of the bioethical standards, apart from the context, provide what is necessary to securely guide Yvonne's response.

THE SCOPE OF THE CONTEXT

In ethics everything is contextual; and the context of every action is unique and unduplicable, with the result that even a small difference between two situations may yield a difference in our moral verdict (Hospers, 1972, p. 63).

Driving 55 miles per hour in a 55-mile per hour zone is ordinarily quite justifiable. It is not justifiable if the road is covered with ice. What is and what is not justifiable entirely depends upon the context.

Dilemma 2-2   Martin is a home health nurse for the Visiting Nurses' Association. He has been caring for Frank for 9 months. Frank has severe chronic obstructive pulmonary disease (COPD). He is rushed into the hospital every 5 or 6 weeks for severe respiratory distress. Frank is a heavy smoker despite his condition. He is also non-compliant in other aspects of his care, such as diet. Martin is considering asking the physician to discontinue home visits. What are the bioethical ramifications of stopping treatment in this case?

A practice-based system of ethical decision making is one that inspires **objectively** justifiable actions. No noncontextual system is relevant to practice, nor are any objectively justifiable. If a system is to inspire relevant and justifiable actions, it must be oriented to the context in which the action is to take place. Ethical actions are justified by reference to ethical purposes. Ethical purposes are justified by reference to vital, fundamental, and long-term values. An agent's purpose is brought to a situation by the agent. The interweaving of a situation and a purpose forms a context. The facts that are relevant to a purpose—to an agent's decisions and actions—will be found in the situation. These facts and the agent's purposive awareness are the interweaving that brings the context into existence.

Every ethical action has meaningful effects lasting beyond the immediate moment. Otherwise, it would not be an ethical action. Ethical actions are actions taken in the pursuit of vital, fundamental, and long-term goals.

ACHIEVEMENT, LOSS, AND THE CONTEXT

Ethical actions are actions taken in the pursuit of vital and fundamental goals. They are actions intended to make an important difference in a person's life. Ethical action requires an interplay between a person and a situation.

This situation must either offer the person the possibility of achieving some value or it must threaten the loss of some value (Husted & Husted, 1993).

Dilemma 2-3   Mrs. Allison, a 56-year-old Australian woman, was admitted to Outback Hospital in critical condition. On report, Josh, Mrs. Allison's nurse, takes note of the fact that she has gotten worse on the 3-11 shift, and decides to make her the first patient he visits after report. He assesses Mrs. Allison and decides that, in his opinion (he considers himself an expert practitioner), she is extremely critical and needs to have more aggressive treatment done quickly. He is aware that his hospital does not have the means to give her the treatment that she needs, but that another urban hospital about 30 miles away does.

The policy at Outback is that an attending physician must sign a transfer order. The attending physician cannot be reached. Since

Outback is a small, rural hospital, there are no interns or residents and no physicians are at the hospital. It is around midnight. Josh would have tried to convince another physician to break policy and sign the transfer order since Mrs. Allison's condition is worsening, but this it not an option. Josh cannot convince anyone in nursing administration to risk going against the policy. What, given his context of knowledge, should he do?

THE INTERWEAVING OF CONTEXTS

The context of the situation is a context of discovery. Through the context of the situation, an agent discovers whether something ought to be done, what ought to be done, and for whom it ought to be done. The context of knowledge is primarily a context of justification. Through the context of knowledge, an agent discovers how it should be done.

A context is very much like a sweater. All the strands making up a sweater are interwoven. Likewise, all the facts, ideas, and beliefs making up a context are interwoven. The interweaving of a sweater is what keeps the strands together and makes it a sweater. The interweaving of the strands of a context is, likewise, that which keeps it together and makes it a context.

A context is the interweaving of three things:

1. The situation a person faces insofar as the situation is related to his desires, purposes, and actions. A situation is a group of related facts. The group of facts that form the context are those facts that can assist or hinder the desires, purposes, and actions of the person dealing with them.

2. The ideas that structure the person's awareness of the facts is the context of his knowledge. This awareness is an awareness of the situation, the action he might take, and of how the situation will assist or hinder his purposes and actions.

3. The ideas and attitudes that an agent brings to the situation.

Efficient ethical decision making requires an interweaving of the context of knowledge into the context of the situation in a way that leads to an appropriate insight.

On any given day, in order for a person to decide whether she ought to wear a coat to go outside, she must have a preexisting body of knowledge. She ought to know, in general, which weather conditions call for a coat. She must determine what the actual weather conditions are outside at this time. It is desirable for her to determine what changes in the weather are in store. Whether she will wear a coat is her dilemma. Knowing what weather conditions, in general, mandate the wearing of a coat is the preexisting part of her context of knowledge. It is that part that she brings to the situation. The weather conditions as they are outside right now is the context of this specific situation.

Her awareness of these conditions is that part of her context of knowledge that she acquires directly from the situation.

In the form of a syllogism, the decision would be made like this:

Whenever it is below 40° F, I ought to wear a coat (context of knowledge).

It is now below 40° F (context of the situation).

Therefore, I ought to wear a coat.

This decision is based on an interweaving of the context of the situation into the context of the agent's knowledge. It is a logically justifiable decision.

A nurse, in her role as such, must be aware of changes in her patient's condition. In the same way, a nurse, in her role as ethical agent, must be aware of changes in the ethical context.

Knowledge of ethical principles is an inner resource that an agent brings to a situation. A systematic awareness of this resource is necessary if it is to function beneficially. An agent's awareness must make it possible for her to analyze that which is known in a logical, step-by-step process. The analysis enables a decision maker to view the situation as an intelligible whole. An agent seeing the situation as an intelligible whole, relevant to her decisions, is seeing it as a context.

Purposes determine contexts. Awareness of her purpose enables an agent to interweave the elements of the situation and, thereby, act in an optimally appropriate way. Attention to the context enables a decision maker to act with maximum efficiency in bringing about a desired outcome. It can enable a nurse to act with maximum efficiency in laying the groundwork to help her patient to arrive at the best decision for him to make at any point in time.

A decision made out of context can never, except through pure chance, be a correct decision. Without attention to the context, there is no way to know whether the decision is most likely to bring about the most desirable result—whether it is ethically justifiable. Regardless of how well an ethical agent understands the logical interconnections of abstract ethical concepts, outside of the context there is no way to know whether a decision is appropriate to the context.

The Context of the Situation

The agent's context of knowledge, including her awareness of relevant principles of judgement, enables her to recognize the context of the situation. The context of the situation provides the criteria that guide her in the application of the ethical principles. Attention to the aspects of the situation that are relevant to her purposes makes it possible for an agent to relate her ethical actions to her ethical purposes.

If an ethical agent were to take actions without reference to the context of the situation, the situation would be irrelevant to her actions. Her actions would also be irrelevant in relation to the situation. Her actions would be unintelligible and purposeless.

For this reason, a discussion of ethical issues in isolation from a context can never lead to a meaningful ethical insight. Issues are, of necessity, disjointed, and unrelated to real-life situations or to each other.

When issues in isolation form a context, the context is sufficient only to lead a nurse to a predetermined conclusion. For this reason, discussions of ethical issues often serve, not to strengthen and expand a nurse's knowledge, but to harden her prejudices. She is thrown back on the nebulous ethical notions that she has acquired, without analysis, through random cultural influences. It is possible to discuss issues such as organ transplantation, abortion, euthanasia, the use of fetal tissue, genetic engineering, treatment of anencephalic infants, and human experimentation, and come away fundamentally uninfluenced by the discussion and with nothing to apply to a real-life dilemma.

The context of a situation is those aspects of the situation that enable a health care professional to identify its nature—what the situation is and what it is not. The aspects of the situation relate to the purposes of the people acting in it. To act according to the context of the situation means to act with awareness of the human purposes that make the situation important as an object of attention. This requires awareness of the ethical resources that can be brought to bear to serve life, health, and well-being. Purposes produce causal processes, and the stronger the purposes, the clearer the causal processes. The more obvious it is that events are the result of the causal actions of interacting agents and the effects of their actions, the more intelligible the context. The more difficult it is to perceive the purposes that motivate actions and the relationship between causes and effects, the less intelligible the context will be.

Her awareness of causal processes in the context makes it possible for a professional to guide her actions according to that which is implied by the situation in relation to her ethical and professional purposes. Without an awareness of the context of the situation, she has no reason to act—and cannot act with reason. Awareness of the ethical situation is the foundation of a practice-based, relevant ethic. Unless the causal processes forming the context of the situation are perceived, no ethical action is possible. "[T]he perceptual grasp of a situation is context dependent, that is, the subtle changes take on significance only in light of the patient's past history and current situation" (Benner, 1984, p. 5).

A nurse's maintaining awareness of the context of the situation while she is acting means her maintaining an awareness of the agreements and responsibilities that structure her ethical situation. It also means her maintaining an awareness of changes in those contextual factors that must shape her actions if she is to act effectively.

Tina has promised to take a group of chronically ill pediatric patients to the zoo. Her purpose is to share their enjoyment. The children—their desires and

their handicaps—form the essential context of the situation. While Tina is preparing for the trip, she discovers that Brucie, the sickest of the children, is scheduled for surgery the next day and will not be able to go on the trip.

Tina is not motivated by a sense of duty. Nor is she devoted to the greatest good for the greatest number. This change in the situation causes her to cancel the trip. She would not enjoy the trip knowing that Brucie could not come with them. She hopes the children would not want to go without Brucie and will be content to wait until later for the trip.

Tina maintained an awareness of the context. This enabled her to be aware of a change in the context and the influence this change had on her purpose. Then, however, Tina discovered another fact in the situation—a fact that changed the context of the situation for her again. She discovered that Brucie was afraid of animals and really did not want to go to the zoo. So Tina explained the situation (less than the entire truth) to the children. Brucie was spared an embarrassing moment, and everyone had a wonderful time at the zoo.

The Context of Knowledge

The context of the situation provides a person with an awareness that there is something to be done. In conjunction with her knowledge of her patient's purposes, it provides her with an awareness of what is to be done. "Keeping the context" is the act of maintaining an awareness of the factors relevant to her ethical actions and changes in these factors. Keeping the context is the first order of ethical action. The context must shape a person's actions if she is to act effectively.

The fact that there is a situation accessible to the purposes of an agent is not enough for the existence of a context. There must be an agent whose knowledge enables her to recognize the nature of the situation. In addition, she must have a desire to act within the situation. She must see it as either requiring action to prevent some undesirable consequence or possessing aspects necessary to the accomplishment of a desirable goal.

This awareness (knowledge) on the part of an agent presupposes that she is able to put the relevant aspects of the situation together into an intelligible form. This is what a nurse does, for instance, each time she makes a nursing diagnosis.

Every decision that an agent makes, if she acts "in (or according to) the context" must be made according to:

- Her knowledge
- That which is relevant in the situation

Her knowledge enables her to recognize what is relevant in the situation. That which is relevant in the situation enables her to apply her knowledge. Both together enable her to act to accomplish her purposes.

An agent's context of knowledge includes her awareness of those aspects of the situation that invite action. Her awareness of the possibilities for success in alternative courses of action is also part of her context of knowledge.

An agent's keeping the context of her knowledge involves an awareness of changes in her knowledge, an awareness of the emergence of new factors that threaten the realization of her purposes, that offer new ways of realizing them, or that offer new values worthy of pursuit.

In reference to ethical decision making, a context of knowledge is both a body of prior knowledge and a state of present awareness. A nurse's ethical knowledge and awareness must be relevant to the attainment of fundamental, vital, and long-term goals. Otherwise, what purpose would ethical knowledge have? The knowledge of a decision maker—an agent acting for her own interests in relation to the circumstances in which she acts—is the context of her knowledge. Where she acts as the agent of another—as a health care professional acts as the agent of her patient—the ethical knowledge she brings to the situation and her awareness of the ethical aspects of the situation is, once again, the context of her knowledge.

A CHANGE OF DIRECTION

An ethical decision is one that:

- We are going to act upon (it is more than theorizing).
- Will guide our actions.
- Will give us a reason to believe that our actions will make life better.
- Actually affects our life over a considerable span of time.
- Will enable us to change our directions as we act upon it.

This last point is especially important. There is a difference between being able to change the direction of actions when the direction proves to be mistaken and being tied into a course of action and not having the power to change it. This difference makes a difference in whatever we do in our lives.

Two things follow from this: A nurse has a responsibility to interact with a patient as a person—as one human being with another. A professional acts best when she remembers that she is a human being; her patient is a human being; and she acts as one human being with another.

A professional has a responsibility to interact with patients in order to assist them to avoid failures and to bring about their successes.

Human beings can make mistakes. A human being can make a decision and come to realize that she has made the wrong decision. When this happens, there are two things she can do:

1. She can make herself unconscious and refuse to let herself know that her decision is a bad one.
2. She can change her direction.

REASONING AND DECISION MAKING

There is a **habitual** way of thinking that keeps a person from changing her ethical decisions and her actions. This always causes chaos and misery. The worst part is that when we form this habit, we are very seldom aware of adopting it. But many people, too late, have discovered that their personal tragedy was caused by this way of thinking. And many never discover it.

This way of thinking involves the difference between reasoning **to** a decision and reasoning **from** a decision.

If you reason **to** a decision, you start with objective reality—what is out there in the health care setting—your patient's world.

If you reason **from** a decision, you start from you own subjectivity—from your present unquestioned beliefs—and from your feelings.

Two examples of reasoning to a decision are: "As a nurse, what should my ethical attitude toward my profession be?" "What can I learn from my patients?"

Two examples of reasoning from a decision are: "As a nurse, how am I going to go about forcing my beliefs onto the health care setting?" "What can my patients learn from me?"

The difference is in where you begin. If you begin with facts out there in the world, you can make a decision based on what you discover out in the world. If you begin with the fact that the efficient practice of your profession calls for a specific and consistent ethical attitude—and that it is your task to create it—you will be reasoning from the objective facts **to** a decision. This is beginning from an objective perspective.

If you begin with your feelings, or the way things **seem** to you, or decisions that you made in the past, and you refuse to look at facts **here and now**, you will be reasoning **from** a decision that is already made—and trying to rationalize that decision. This is beginning from a subjective perspective: "I am indifferent to the ethical foundation of my profession. I will think of excuses on the spur of the moment." The worst part of this is, if you do begin here, you may never get out of the subjective perspective into the realities of your profession.

THE ABANDONED CONTEXT

Imagine that you live on an island. This island is ruled by a disoriented and ill-directed king. The king of the island is passionately interested in increasing

the happiness and contentment of his subjects. This poses a serious threat to them. At this time, there are exactly 100 inhabitants on the island. A panel of experts has informed the king that 10 of his subjects are the happiest and most contented 10% on the island. Another 10 are in the 90th percentile, and so on down to the unhappiest and most discontented 10% of the population.

The king reasons that without this unhappiest 10% of the population, the society he rules would be, statistically, happier. Accordingly, the king has the 10 least happy citizens of his island kingdom drowned.

Now, assuming you were not one of the unhappy 10, let us continue. When this statistically unhappy 10% is disposed of, the island society, on a mathematical basis, is about 5.5% happier and more contented. At the same time, you will notice, your mood is entirely unchanged. It is the same with everyone on the island. Not one individual is happier or more contented by an eyelash. A disinterested observer might discover a number of flaws in the king's decision-making process:

1. A context can enable a person to begin to solve an ethical dilemma. It cannot, by itself, serve to solve the dilemma. The king assumed that the dilemma, in effect, solved itself. He applied no ethical principles to the context. He simply observed the context and applied a mathematical equation.

2. The king was not aware of the difference between the nature of a group of 100 individual women and men and the nature of a single individual woman or man.

This is the central reason why he failed to solve the dilemma he perceived. He failed to maintain the context of his knowledge. Before a person becomes a king—or an ethical agent—he should know the difference between a percentage and a person. The king did not maintain an awareness of the difference between concrete realities (the individual women and men who lived on the island) and mental abstractions (the percentages studied by his panel of experts).

3. He failed to maintain the context of the situation. If there are two people on an island and one dies, the sum of his happiness will not accrue to the other. His death may very well diminish the happiness of the other. What holds true of two people, in this context, holds true of a hundred. The king's action was entirely irrational. In order to maintain the context, a person must differentiate between the rational and the irrational. The king did not.

4. The king did not maintain an awareness of simple causal factors. There are values that make people happy and contented, and losses that make them unhappy and discontented. Other people on the island had died without their deaths influencing the happiness or unhappiness of the entire citizenry. There is nothing in the nature of individual people or happiness or death such that the death of the unhappy increases the happiness of the living.

5.   The king kept himself unaware of the nature of a fundamental, interpersonal, ethical concept. He maintained an unawareness of the rights of his subjects. The rights to autonomy, individual freedom, and self-assertion cannot be the rights of a percentage. All rights are the rights of individuals.

The king kept himself unaware of the fact that rights accrue to people because of their human nature. The belief that a person loses his right to life when he becomes unhappy is absurd. There is nothing in the nature of individual people, of rights, or of happiness to justify this belief.

The king would not have made a good biomedical professional. For him, 100 people as a group is a reality no different from an individual man or woman. No one who cannot differentiate between an individual and a group can make a good king or a good biomedical professional.

Ethics, and especially bioethics, has to do with individuals. Health care dilemmas are, essentially, dilemmas concerning individual clinicians and patients. The context is interpersonal and individual—a context involving two interacting individuals. It is not a solitary context. But neither is it a group or a statistical context.

ETHICAL INDIVIDUALISM AND THE LAW

The distinction between the law and ethics is that the law is external to the person, while ethics is internal to the person. The law is concerned with the whole of society as opposed to the individual. Ethics is concerned with the good of the individual (Guido, 1997).

Every patient who enters the health care system, concerned for his survival and well-being, enters as an ethical individualist. Many lawsuits have originated over the failure of the health care system to recognize this. Virtually every law that relates to these issues sanctions the patient's ethical individualism.[4] The law recognizes (among other things):

- A patient's legal right to give an informed consent. No one has a legal right to treat a patient without his consent. No one has a legal right to obtain a patient's consent without the patient's knowing to what he is giving his consent.
- A patient's legal right to refuse treatment.
- A patient's legal right, postmortem, to be protected against the "harvesting" of organs.
- The legal right of children to medical attention regardless of the wishes of their parents.
- A patient's legal right to confidentiality.
- An individual's legal right to refuse to donate organs (e.g., bone marrow) to a relative.

- A patient's legal right not to participate in research against his wishes.
- A patient's legal right to be protected against malpractice or wrongful death.

Each of these rights had to be recognized as an ethical right before it was enacted as a legal right.

THE NECESSARY, THE SUFFICIENT, AND THE ETHICAL

Let us pause to examine a crucial aspect of ethical reality through a thought experiment.

Your son shows the symptoms of a physical disorder, leading you to take him to a pediatrician. The pediatrician examines him and tells you, "Your son will have to have a nephrectomy." Stunned, you leave the pediatrician's office and stop in a nearby coffee shop. In a few moments, the pediatrician comes in and you beckon him over. A remarkable conversation takes place.

You ask the pediatrician, "If my son undergoes a nephrectomy, will this be sufficient for his recovery?" The pediatrician replies, "No, in all honesty, I cannot say that the operation alone will bring about his recovery. The operation, in itself, will not be sufficient to bring your son back to good health."

You continue to question the pediatrician by asking him, "Is this operation a necessary part of my son's recovery? Would it be possible to bring him back to health without the operation?" The pediatrician replies, "Well, yes. There are other ways to treat him that will bring about an optimum recovery. The nephrectomy is not a necessary mode of treatment. In fact, the nephrectomy is neither sufficient in itself to return your son to health, nor is it necessary for his recovery."

You smile and rise. You express your pleasure at having met the pediatrician. You turn, breathe a sigh of relief, herd your son through the door, and, needless to say, you never visit this pediatrician again.

If one thing is neither necessary nor sufficient to bring about a second thing, it has no significant causal relation to the second thing (Mill, 1843). If a nephrectomy is neither necessary nor sufficient to the recovery of your son, it is entirely useless and irrelevant in relation to your son's treatment and recovery.

Let us examine how the necessary and the sufficient plays out in bioethics.

If an ethical approach provides what is necessary, and an agent wants to succeed at ethical interaction, then she should follow this approach. It is necessary to her ethical action, which means that her ethical interactions cannot succeed without it.

If it is sufficient and more desirable (more certain to bring about a desired outcome, less apt to go out of control and bring about an undesirable outcome) than any other way of directing her actions, then she ought to adopt it in preference to a different approach.

If it is both necessary and sufficient then, by all means, an agent ought to adopt it. Since it is necessary, she cannot succeed without it. Since it is sufficient, nothing else is necessary.

If an ethical approach is neither necessary nor sufficient, if it will not enable an agent to succeed at ethical interaction, and if her ethical interaction can succeed without it, then it is of no use to her. There is no reason for her to adopt it.

Utilitarianism is not sufficient to produce effective and justifiable ethical interaction.

Utilityville is a village run on utilitarian principles. Periodically, the town fathers randomly choose someone to serve the community. They put this person in chains in the public square and torture him to death. They inflict a punishment on this innocent person similar but milder to that which they would inflict on a habitual criminal.

The death of this unfortunate benefactor serves the community in two ways:

1. Once they witness the gruesome fate of an entirely innocent person, potential criminals can imagine, in bloodcurdling detail, the horrible fate awaiting the guilty. This leads a number of potential criminals away from a life of crime and a horrible death by torture. This, in itself, brings about "the greatest good for the greatest number."

But it has even further benefits:

2. Many people who would otherwise be victims of crime are saved from this fate by the death of the village benefactor.

The town fathers are highly motivated to save potential victims of crime. They have found a very effective way to bring about "the greatest good for the greatest number." They save potential victims by making actual victims.

There is a drawback to this practice. It violates any rational conception of justice. This type of crime prevention must produce intolerable conditions. These conditions cannot be made right by more utilitarianism. There is nothing in utilitarianism to prevent any crime by a greater number against a lesser number or against an individual. Individual justice is necessary to a human form of existence and to objectively justifiable ethical action. Nothing in the principle of utility[5] establishes the principle of individual justice. The recognition of individual rights must be added to the principle of utility in the attempt to prevent barbaric acts of injustice.

Utilitarianism alone is not sufficient to rationally justifiable ethical interaction.

In Utilityville, the practice of utilitarianism is not necessary to effective and justifiable ethical action. Such action would be quite possible without it. Societies based on individual rights, nonaggression, and interaction through agreement flourish far better than utilitarian societies.

It is clear that utilitarianism is not necessary to rational, ethical interaction.

As an ethical approach, utilitarianism is neither sufficient in itself nor a necessary addition to other approaches to bring about justifiable ethical action.

No health care setting should be a Utilityville. Utility undermines a professional's ethical awareness by directing her away from the objectives of her profession. **Deontology** fares no better than utilitarianism.

If a person marooned on a desert island were to pursue duties rather than the needs of her survival, her actions might well be regarded as pathological. If she were to conceive of the pursuit of her survival as a duty, it would do nothing whatever to strengthen her efforts. In fact, it would impede her efforts. Few things inspire a greater determination than the pursuit of one's survival in a grave situation, while duties tend to the nature of the unpleasant, undesirable, and burdensome.

In an interpersonal situation, the principle would be the same. For a deontologist, it is not the reasonableness of interaction that justifies either the action or the deontologist as agent. It is his action in following his duty, taken in isolation from the quality or the consequences of his action. Deontology does not produce intelligible ethical interactions. It is an understatement to say that deontology is not sufficient to bring about objectively justifiable ethical interaction.

In an interpersonal context, the pursuit of duty would be a threat to survival. It would inhibit rational, ethical action. The establishment of a slave society, the pursuit of genocide, and the destruction of medical science are all actions compatible with deontology. Again, individual rights, nonaggression, and interaction through agreement are necessary to rational human interaction.[6]

Deontology is not a self-sufficient approach, nor is deontology necessary to bring about rational and effective ethical interaction.

Imagine a society in which the individual members were inspired by the idea of individual rights. Aggression is foreign to the folkways of this society. All interaction occurs through mutual agreement. Deontology would add nothing of value to this society. It would undermine the recognition of individual rights. It would conflict with the idea of interaction through agreement.

Nonaggression is to a society what health is to an individual. Deontology is perfectly compatible with aggression. A recognition of individual rights is the royal road to nonaggression. There is nothing that could be added to deontology that would make it practical in any society. If that which is added is beneficial, it does not need the support of duty. If it is harmful, duty will not make it beneficial.

Deontology is neither sufficient nor necessary to rational and justifiable ethical interaction. It undermines ethical thinking in the health care setting. It makes **living** a profession impossible.

RELEVANCE AND A PRACTICE-BASED ETHIC

The case with bioethics is very different. A practice-based bioethics is both necessary and sufficient to optimally effective ethical action in a biomedical setting.

Symphonia is a Greek word meaning agreement. **Symphonology** is the study of agreements. For the purpose of this book, it is the study of agreements in the health care arena among health care professionals and patients.

A **symphonological** ethic—a practice-based ethic structured on agreement—creates intelligibility in the relationship and interaction between the professional and her patient. In the health care setting, a nurse's role is intelligible to her. A patient's condition makes him aware of his role. These facts produce the agreement that makes for the intelligibility and harmony of their relationship.

The nurse/patient agreement establishes intelligibility by means of a shared understanding of the purposes and ground rules of their relationship and interaction. This understanding is the only possible rational ground of effective ethical interaction.

The professional/patient agreement and its implications are necessary to intelligible and effective ethical interaction (as discussed in chapter 4). The bioethical standards are all implied by the nurse/patient agreement (as discussed in chapter 5).

The understanding between nurse and patient requires, on some level of awareness, a recognition of the bioethical principles. A certain level of awareness is necessary in order for the agreement to be made. This awareness must include awareness of the bioethical principles. A recognition of the principles as ethical guidelines within the agreement, as we will see, is both necessary and sufficient to a practice-based ethic. Such an ethic objectively assures the most efficient cooperation possible between nurse and patient.

The traditional ethical approaches will not produce efficient bioethical interaction. Therefore, a practice-based professional ethic is **necessary** and **sufficient** to efficient ethical interaction. A practice-based ethic maximally enhances the ambience and the efficiency of the health care setting. It reveals what is possible to the health care setting.

CONTEXTUAL CERTAINTY

While persons seek certainty in their decisions, "... moral [ethical] certainty can provide [unwarranted] comfort for the ethical decision maker ... and stifle dialogue and in-depth discussion of the [situation]" (Wurzbach, 1999, p. 287). Wurzbach goes on to say that when nurses "feel" too certain of their decisions, they tend not to question their own beliefs and actions, do not dialogue with themselves, and do not look for possible alternatives to their actions so mistakes can be avoided. They overlook the possibilities of "gentle coercion." (For a brief discussion of gentle coercion, please see the glossary.)

The only possible ethical certainty a person can have in a biomedical setting is contextual certainty, which is possible to a limited time and a specific circumstance.

Certainty is only possible to the extent that:

1. One has relevant facts available as evidence pointing toward a decision—the context of the situation.
2. One has relevant knowledge to apply to these facts—a context of knowledge. An attempt to escape awareness of the situation, or to evade one's **knowledge**, cannot change this. Irrelevance is not a solution to the problem of certainty (Husted & Husted, 1998, p. 238).

THE WISDOM OF SHERLOCK HOLMES

> "The most important truths conceal themselves behind the most obvious facts."
>
> (Doyle, 1930)

The ethics committee from Cyber-space Hospital are presented with a dilemma. A young man, Greg, has been admitted into the hospital with a broken leg suffered during a boating accident. At this time in the hospital, there are two patients needing a corneal transplant, two patients needing a kidney transplant, a patient needing a liver transplant, and another needing a heart transplant. As luck would have it, Greg is a match for all six of these patients. The committee rejects the suggestion that Greg's organs be harvested for the benefit of the transplant candidates. It is an obvious fact that this is an irrational suggestion.

Yet why is it irrational? If we all have a duty to assist others, the young man then has multiple duties to donate his organs. Also, this course of action would certainly serve the greatest good for the greatest number.

But it is an obvious fact that the course of action suggested cannot be justified ethically. A crucially important ethical truth conceals itself behind this obvious fact. Consider this:

Dilemma 2-4   Harold has a gangrenous leg. Harold's physician wants to perform an amputation in order to save Harold's life. He refuses the surgery. His physician tells him, "No one could possibly want this." She gets a court order declaring Harold incompetent. The court order permits her to perform the surgery. Harold's physician tells herself that she has acted benevolently. At the same time, she has violated Harold's autonomy.

WHAT WOULD HAPPEN IF . . . ?

Few bioethics texts make the human values of those engaged in health care interaction the central focus of their concern. All give some attention to the values and well-being of patients. None hold the health care professional as the primary beneficiary of bioethical interaction. This would be the focus of a rational self-interest ethic.

Rational Self-Interest

The rationality of a rational self-interest ethic begins in its rejection of self-abandonment as the only possible approach to a profession. It equally rejects deception or coercion as the basis of interaction. Rational interaction is conducted on the basis of objective understanding, self-respect, agreement, and fidelity. It cannot be conducted on the basis of unexamined emotions, self-doubt, or the desire to evade responsibility.

A nurse (by definition) is the agent of a patient doing for a patient what he would do for himself if he were able (chapter 3 contains a detailed discussion of the nature of a nurse and her relationship to patients). A patient needs a rational agent to do for him what he would do for himself; simply because what he would do for himself needs to be rational.

A self-interest ethic is practiced by an ethical agent with a view to enhance her life through interaction based on objective agreements—a trade of values—agreements from which she benefits (the function of agreement is covered in detail in Chapter 4).

An agent's rational self-interest is defined in terms of her understanding of her individual nature against the background of what is needed for her personal development. It also requires a complete acceptance of the nature, motivations, and self-interest of her"trading partner."

The functioning of a rational self-interest ethics is well formulated by William Shakespeare in these famous words:

> This above all: to thine own self be true,
> And it must follow, as the night the day,
> Thou canst not then be false to any man.
> (Hamlet, Act I, Scene I)

In this, as in a multitude of things, Shakespeare seems to go too far—but he does not. He is "right on the money."

To be true to oneself one must know oneself and respect oneself.

Let us conduct a little experiment in thought and examine the foreseeable consequences of a nurse practicing according to a rational self-interest ethic.

A nurse's rational self-interest is achieved through the ethical competence of her professional behavior. It is expressed by satisfaction in the practice of her profession, by confidence in her competence to act, in the pride she takes in herself and her professional activities, her feelings of self-contentment—above all in her pride in her ethical ambition. All of this grows out of her professional actions and her assurance that these actions are appropriate to her profession. It arises from her skill at the practice—and the spirit—of her profession. Every nurse begins her career with a decision that she will be a nurse. When she reaches this decision, she assumes that, in some way, her self-interest will be achieved in nursing. Her true self-interest is not served—it is lost the day she decides that her self-interest conflicts with that of her patients (the unsuspected values that a nurse can achieve through nursing is addressed in chapter 9).

Conflicts and the Realities of Nursing

There is one defining fact about nursing that is often ignored. It serves as the foundation of a practice-based bioethic. This fact is that: **A nurse takes no actions that are not interactions.** Every professional action that a nurse takes, is an interaction between herself and a patient. This is true of a professional in the clinical setting. It is equally true, in more complex ways, of nursing administrators, researchers, and educators. To be "true to her own self" for a nurse, so long as she is a nurse, is to be true to her interactions.

The quality of a professional's actions cannot be judged in isolation. It is intrinsically interwoven with, and determined by, the quality of her patient's responses. **A nurse's actions cannot succeed if her patient's responses fail and she could have inspired him to succeed.**

The quality of action is produced by the quality of the virtues that produced it. The quality of interaction is produced by the interlaced virtues of those who interact.

In the context of a rational self-interest ethic, a professional's essential ethical responsibility is to encourage and strengthen her patient's virtues. His virtues are the qualities of his character by which he serves his life, health, and well-being—his power to act in the service of his flourishing and happiness. It is his power to act in the service of **her** professional values—if these values are a reflection of her caring—her personal interest in what happens to him. These virtues are one aspect of the bioethical standards (for an extensive discussion of virtue see chapter 9).

If agreement is fundamental to every aspect of the nurse/patient interaction (and it is), then that which makes agreement possible and interaction successful is the highest professional value. It is the virtues signified by the bioethical standards that make agreement possible and desirable (chapter 5 discusses the bioethical standards in relationship to decision making in detail).

A patient's **autonomy refers to the uniqueness of the individual person. His uniqueness is the specific nature—the motivations and character-structures—of this person.** This virtue involves his self-awareness. It is a nurse's task to clarify and strengthen her patient's autonomy. Only a unique human individual can make agreements. And the form of his agreements is shaped by his uniqueness. A patient needs a self-awareness that is life-serving.

A patient's **freedom is his natural power, and his right, to take long-term actions based on his own awareness of the situation in which he acts.** This virtue is essential to the forming of agreements and the efficacy of a patient's actions. As an ethical right it is his right to live his life. It is a nurse's ethical responsibility to maximize her patient's freedom.

A patient's **objectivity is his need, and his power, to achieve and sustain the exercise of his objective awareness.** It is her task to interact on the basis of the virtue of objective awareness—his and her own.

To the extent that objective awareness is not possible, an agreement is flawed, at best, and, at worst, simply illusory. Even in the case of a patient who cannot engage on the basis of objective awareness, e.g., a comatose patient, objectivity, on the part of a professional, is still necessary—if anything, more necessary than it would be otherwise. Objectivity is the *sine qua non* of successful interaction.

The virtue of a patient's ethical **self-assertion is his power and right to control his time and effort.** It is an implication of his innate nature and powers. It is her responsibility to act for him and, where possible, to enable him to act to maximize his control of his time and effort. No agreement can be formed without the ability to expend time and effort in carrying it out. His self-assertion is the virtue that begins his interaction. The other virtues deliver the momentum to sustain it.

Beneficence, in relation to a patient, is his power and right to act to acquire the benefits he desires, and the needs his life requires. This is the motivation of every agreement. It is her task to expand and heighten his sense of beneficence to strengthen this virtue.

If a person had no rational interest in seeking to achieve benefit and avoid harm (a condition that does not apply to human beings regardless of their age or condition), there would be no occasion for her to be concerned with agreements. Beneficence, the pursuit of benefits, is a precondition of agreement, and the focal point of successful interaction.

The virtue of a patient's **fidelity is his faithfulness to his autonomy. For a nurse, fidelity is commitment to the responsibilities she has accepted as a nurse.** These obligations are structured by the vital and existential needs of her patient. It is her task to solidify her patient's fidelity to himself, his life, health, and well-being—his human values and his happiness.

In their interaction, her fidelity is to her patient, but her patient's fidelity is to himself. If she is dedicated to nursing, then, her competence and pride are built upon her fidelity. Her rational self-interest is nourished by her ability to inspire a patient's fidelity to himself. This is the source of her success as a nurse.

Nurturing a patient's virtues, and her own, is all that is necessary to objectively justifiable ethical action. More than this, it is all that is possible in perfecting a practice-based ethical interaction with a patient. It is the foundation for a nurse's rational self-interest, and a patient's justified trust.

Through this moral cooperation, in the context of nursing practice, everyone wins.

MUSINGS

Achieving awareness of the context means integrating that which is present in the circumstances into all the relevant knowledge that one possesses. Achieving awareness of the context is, in effect, a process of assimilating the context of the situation into a context of knowledge. Losing awareness of the context means ignoring relevant items of knowledge or relevant aspects of the situation. Losing awareness of the context is the worst possible way to begin a decision-making process. Not having awareness of the context makes it impossible to justify a decision.

When a nurse retains awareness of the bioethical context, she and her patient are most apt to gain the maximum benefit of ethical action. For anyone, in any ethical context, to benefit from ethical action, it is necessary for him to retain a clear awareness of the context. Success follows upon effective action. Effective action follows upon **active** awareness.

"The nurse functions both as a professional and as a human being within a variety of contexts. These contexts influence directly or indirectly the way in which the nurse performs caring tasks" (Gastmans, 1998, p. 126).

NOTES

1.   In an ethical context, agency is the power to initiate action and to sustain the actions necessary to successful living. Generally in any ethical relationship between any two people, each functions as an ethical agent. In a relationship between a nurse and a physician, each functions as an agent. The relationship between a nurse and her patient is quite different. A nurse, by definition, is one who performs the role of agent. To a greater or lesser extent, a nurse becomes the agent of her patient. She does for her patient what he would do for himself if he were able—until he regains his agency.

2.   An agent's preexisting knowledge is that general knowledge that she brings to the situation as opposed to the information that she gains from her experience of the specific factors of the situation. Thus, a nurse's recognition of a patient's right to make and act on decisions is part of her preexisting knowledge.

How that recognition relates to this specific patient will depend upon the character of the patient. A nurse will discover the requirements of her patient's individual freedom by discovering the nature of his values and desires. This she learns from the situation. The knowledge that he has a right to individual freedom is part of her preexisting knowledge. Preexisting means applicable to an ethical context but possessed by an ethical agent prior to experience of a specific context.

3.   Formalism is "rigorous or excessive adherence to recognized forms" (*American Heritage College Dictionary*, 1997). An ethical formalist is one who concentrates entirely on the abstract category into which an action can be placed, without regard for the context or the effects of the action.

The spirit of formalism in deontology is captured in the Latin maxim: "One should tell the truth though the heavens fall." If, in a certain country, there were many rich people and very few poor ones, a Robin Hood who robbed from the poor to give to the rich would be practicing a utilitarian formalism.

4.   This is not to suggest that ethical individualism is desirable and proper because it is sanctioned by the law. Individual rights are not produced by law. **Rather, laws are purposeless and unintelligible if they are not derived from individual rights.** Contemporary medical law is desirable and proper because it is sanctioned by ethical individualism.

5.   The "principle of utility" is "the greatest good for the greatest number."

6.   It might be objected that for individual rights to exist, a duty to respect individual rights must exist. This objection would reveal a very superficial understanding of individual rights. The recognition of rights is based on an agreement, not on a duty.

REFERENCES

American Heritage Dictionary (3rd. ed.). (1997). Boston: Houghton Mifflin.

Benner, P. (1984). *From novice to expert*. Menlo Park, CA: Addison-Wesley.

Doyle, A. C. (1930). *The complete Sherlock Holmes (Vol. II): The hound of the baskervilles*. New York: Doubleday.

Gastmans, C. (1998). Challenges to nursing values in a changing nursing environment. *Nursing Ethics, 5*, 236–245.

Guido, G. W. (1997). *Legal issues* (2nd ed.). Stamford, CT: Appleton & Lange.

Hospers, J. (1972). *Human conduct: Problems of ethics*. New York: Harcourt Brace Jovanovich.

Husted, J. H., & Husted, G. L. (1998). The role of the nurse in ethical decision making. In G. De Loughery (Ed.), *Issues and trends in nursing* (3rd ed., pp. 216–242). St. Louis, MO: Mosby.

Husted, J. H., & Husted, G. L. (1993). Personal and impersonal values in bioethical decision making. *Journal of Home Health Care Practice, 5*(4), 59–65.

Mill, J. S. (1843). *A system of logic*. London: Oxford Press.

Polanyi, M. (1958). *The study of man*. Chicago: The University of Chicago Press.
Polanyi, M., & Prosch, H. (1975). *Meaning*. Chicago: The University of Chicago Press.
Wurzbach, M. E. (1999). Acute care nurses' experiences of moral certainty. *Advanced Nursing, 30*, 287–293.

CHAPTER 3

The Ethical Approach of Professional and Patient in the Health Care Setting

The philosopher Lao Tzu (604 B.C.) (Brown, 1938) has told us that "The longest journey begins with the first step." This is so obvious that we can see it for ourselves. We can hardly avoid seeing it. But it is so obvious that, without Lao Tzu, we might never have noticed the importance of it.

It is also obvious that we can take the first step of a journey in confusion. When we take it in confusion, or from an unthinking and arrogant certainty, it is often in the wrong direction. If it is taken in the wrong direction, at the end of our journey we may find ourselves very far from our destination. If it is an ethical journey, we may be unaware of this.

A series of actions taken in the pursuit of vital and fundamental goals may be regarded as an ethical journey. The possibility of arriving at an undesirable destination is very true of an ethical journey.

THE APPROPRIATE AND THE JUSTIFIABLE

Some ethical decisions are appropriate. At the same time, the way they are made is unjustifiable. The agent who makes them does so for a reason. There is a likelihood that they will accomplish their purposes. While accomplishing this purpose, they will injure neither the agent nor anyone else. Often they are made on the basis of hunches and intuitions. They may, nevertheless, by accident, be appropriate to the context in which they are made. But nothing is learned from them and no skills are developed. They are not repeatable. The agent really did not know why she did what she did.

Some ethical decisions are justifiable. They are appropriate to the contexts in which they are made. They accomplish the purposes of the agent and injure no one. That they will bring about some benefit and avoid bringing about harm is foreseeable by the agent who makes them. The acting agent can see, like a causal chain, the connections between her decision, the actions she takes, and the results of her actions. She knows why she made this decision. If it were necessary, she could explain and justify her motives to an objective observer. Before she took her ethical action, she explained and justified her motives to herself. Since she, herself, is an objective observer, she has made a justifiable decision.

THE UNJUSTIFIABLE

Any ethical decision that is justifiable must be appropriate to the context in which it was made. Otherwise, it would not be justifiable. One cannot, in any logical sense, justify an inappropriate ethical decision. One cannot establish appropriateness outside of a context. That an ethical decision is justifiable presupposes that it is appropriate—at least to the decision maker's context of knowledge.

But an (apparently) appropriate ethical decision is not necessarily justifiable:

- The agent may not be able to explain her motivations. She may not be clearly aware of her motivations.
- She may be unable to give a description that explains the causal connections between her motivations and her decision.
- She may be unable to give a description explaining the predictable connections between her decision and the accomplishment of her purpose.
- She may not have a clear and coherent knowledge of why her decisions are appropriate to the circumstances under which she made them.

Ethical decisions made under these conditions are not justifiable by the nurse who makes them. Her action may have been successful, but she had no clear vision of its purpose or outcome.

Dilemma 3-1   An ambulance has brought Mr. Nathan into the hospital. He is vomiting and complaining about severe pain in his abdomen. The physician examines him and makes a preliminary diagnosis of appendicitis. The blood work confirms this diagnosis. Mr. Nathan refuses to undergo surgery. The surgeon asks Mr. Nathan's nurse, Anthony, to get Mr. Nathan's consent. What should Anthony do?

Mr. Dietrich is hospitalized. All his desires and intentions have been interrupted. As with every human being, the processes of thought, choice, decision, and action are natural to Mr. Dietrich. But now he cannot translate thought into action.

Mr. Dietrich's power of agency is nullified, and all his purposeful and goal-directed actions are frustrated. To seek values and to arrange these values into a more perfect life is natural to all humans. But Mr. Dietrich can only seek to rid himself of disvalues.

Mr. Dietrich expects beneficence from his nurse. He cannot know, and he probably would not believe, that his nurse would make an ethical decision involving him without her knowing, objectively, **why** that decision was made. To do so would be a failure of beneficence. Mr. Dietrich, like every patient, assumes beneficence on the part of his nurse.

Mr. Dietrich is in the final stages of cancer. He probably will not live out the week. His physician has ordered physical therapy for him. Mr. Dietrich does not want to go to therapy. His nurse assumes that the physician has some reason for the therapy and decides that she will not question his decision.

Can the nurse justify her decision? She has no reason to believe that it was an appropriate decision for the physician to make. In fact, it seems obvious that it is an inappropriate decision—irrelevant, at best, to Mr. Dietrich's circumstances. Physicians do make inappropriate decisions based on facts irrelevant to a patient's values and circumstances.[1]

Mr. Dietrich would have no reason to imagine that his nurse has no clear awareness of the relationship between the decision to make him endure the pain of therapy and the purposes that are appropriate to his context.

There is no **ethical** justification for Mr. Dietrich's nurse to remain unaware. Yet, all too often, ethical decisions suffer this sort of defect. We all know this. But we do not like to think about it. All the same, a nurse has an ethical responsibility to think about it.

Generally, a nurse will learn from experience what is to be done. But no one can function well without an open and clear awareness of what she is doing and why she is doing it. In addition, the nurse's role is difficult. Her environment is filled with distractions. Even under conditions that make justifiable ethical decisions impossible, a nurse can make appropriate ethical decisions, although not with perfect assurance, serenity, or consistency.

Justifiable ethical decision making is not impossible. It is not even difficult in most situations. But it is impossible solely on the basis of hunches and intuitions. It is also impossible on the basis of tradition or laws. These " . . . imply a psychology of moral motivation in which anxiety and dependence are the primary [ethical] motivators" (van Hooft, 1990, p. 210).

In the final analysis, the emphasis for bioethics is not on what a nurse ought to do but on her character. As Tunna and Conner (1993) have said of nurses:

> . . . a degree of misdirection exists in contemporary nursing ethics. The focus is almost exclusively on what nurses ought to do with little emphasis on how the nurses, themselves, should be. Consequently, practitioners may believe that character is not an issue and that doing the right thing (according to rules predetermined by others) is what matters (pp. 25–26).

PREPARING FOR THE ETHICAL JOURNEY

If a health care professional can develop the ability to objectively justify ethical decisions, she has, by that very fact, developed the ability to make appropriate decisions. But it seems impossible that she could develop an ability to make appropriate decisions consistently if she does not possess the ability to objectively justify decisions.

In order to develop the ability to make justifiable decisions, she must have a sound ethical orientation toward her role. This must be derived from the nature and purposes of her profession. If she has this orientation, she can begin any ethical journey with calm assurance.

To get the direction precisely right, the initial preparations are very important. These preparations are pivotal in the ethical decision making of any professional. In order to be certain of its discovery, a number of conditions of the search are desirable:

1. The work-a-day world should not be considered. The work-a-day world is a blooming, buzzing confusion. The ethical aspects of a situation are usually so snarled up in logistic and administrative concerns and the demands of "hands on" care that they are obscured.

2. The authentically ethical aspects of a situation should be clearly perceived. It will also be desirable to be able to fill in the details of the health care setting. These details, held in the mind's eye, will keep one in the context of one's profession. But, being only in the mind's eye, they will not interfere with ethical analysis and discovery.

3. The essential qualities of the ethical situation should be visualized. For instance, it is commonly agreed that bioethics calls for a patient's right to self-assertion to be respected. A patient's right to self-assertion can be a fuzzy abstraction. Its outline may become visible only in the most obvious circumstances.

A disoriented patient is being transferred on a gurney. He throws off his covers. The situation almost beckons to the nurse to replace them. However, very few situations are as simple as this.

A cloudy understanding of a patient's right to self-assertion—his right to control his own situation—is better than no ethical understanding at all. But it is better, and far more useful, if a nurse understands that this patient has a right to be protected against undesired or undesirable interaction of any sort. This illustrates self-assertion.

4.   The essential qualities of a situation are those qualities that can, properly, guide the nurse's ethical actions. They are like landmarks on a trip, guiding the traveler to his destination. The ethical aspects of a situation should be isolated. One should be able to draw general—but tentative—conclusions to apply to very similar situations. Without these general conclusions, a nurse has to face similar situations, one by one, without understanding.

5.   It is important to make decisions that have a beneficial effect into the future. It is of little importance to make decisions whose benefits cease the moment the actions are taken. Ethical actions do not have to occur in disjointed series. They can be taken in an ongoing integrated sequence.

An ethical decision maker is very much like a pool player. An unskilled pool player merely attempts to put a ball into a pocket. An unskilled decision maker decides on what **seems** best and acts on it.

A skilled pool player sets up shots and tries to put a ball into a pocket while leaving the cueball in such a position that it will be easy to make the next shot. A skilled decision maker makes decisions purposefully. A skilled nurse makes decisions based on the purposes of the patient and on what is necessary to accomplish them. A skilled decision maker does not exert intense mental effort in order to make arrhythmic ethical decisions, but masters the process of bioethical decision making as a skill. She will not assume that the 'instinctual' behavior that she has been conditioned to by her childhood training is adequate to the health care setting.

6.   Her decisions should be based on stable and permanent values, not on changing and impermanent ones. They should be relevant values, appropriate to a human being in the health care setting. These values, certainly, should be the patient's values and appropriate to the patient at this time. It is better, therefore, to see where these stable and permanent values are than to identify transitory ones.

Suppose an anthropologist from another planet came to earth to study mankind. If he were to understand humans, he would have to be, like humans, an animal organism with the power of reason. He would have to face the same problems and demands for action that humans face. Otherwise, he could not understand human action. Which means that he would be unable to understand human beings.

In order to make his study, he might decide to study the nature of the health care setting. He would discover that, if certain assumptions are made, the health care setting is both intelligible and understandable. But if these assumptions are not made, it is neither.

Through the nature and purposes of the health care setting, he would discover that humans enjoy benefits and suffer harms through unforeseeable events. Then he would discover the following facts about human beings and human life:

- Cooperation is possible and human action is predictable.
- There is a natural benevolence among humans, and trust in the good-will of others is reasonable.
- Integrity and respect for rights is necessary to interaction.
- Foresightful and purposeful interaction based on an exchange of values is possible.

These are the human virtues that make the establishment of a health care setting possible. So long as these virtues direct events in the health care setting, it is intelligible. It produces well-structured ethical values. When they do not, the health care setting becomes a "blooming, buzzing," and morally catastrophic confusion. **The first ethical demand placed on health care professionals is that they recognize the nature, demands, and purposes of the health care setting.** Everything follows from this.

These virtues are assumed when the health care setting is established. But, often, awareness of them is lost. As in many spheres of human action, we abandon the real world and create another world out of empty ethical abstractions. Ethical agents become disoriented through the repetition of words and phrases. Then we live in a world that is created by whim and rationalization (Mahler, Pine, & Bergman, 1975).

THE NATURE OF ETHICAL ASPECTS

Take the sparsest situation imaginable. Imagine two people meeting and beginning to interact in the middle of a wasteland. Not even in this situation is every aspect an ethical aspect. One person plans to follow the North Star and walk out of the wasteland. The other intends to build a fire and lay down debris spelling out "Help" in the hope that a passing airplane will sight him.

Each person has come from different conditions of life. Each has different motivations. Each has different ways of going about things and each will return to different conditions of life. Each has a unique set of abilities, strengths, and weaknesses. The way each has chosen to escape the wasteland is not an ethical aspect of the situation. Neither is the background from which each has come, nor the conditions of life to which they hope to return. Their state of health is not an ethical aspect and neither is their knowledge or lack of knowledge. Taken in itself, their way of approaching problems is not an ethical aspect of the situation. It becomes an ethical aspect only in relation to the situation they actually face.

Every ethical aspect of a situation arises in relation to aspects that are not, in themselves, ethical.

The nonethical aspects of a situation determine what can be done. The ethical aspects—in relation to a purpose—determine what **ought** to be done, given what can be done.

Jane sees a young girl, Nancy, drowning. Jane cannot swim. There is a life preserver at hand. This establishes what Jane can do, but not what Jane ought to do. Jane's ethical character, her sense of beneficence, determines what she ought to do.

Ethics has to do with **actions taken in the pursuit of vital** (essentially related to the preservation or enhancement of life) **and fundamental** (essential to making a person's life what he wants his life to be) **goals.** To rescue Nancy is, at that time, Jane's only vital and fundamental goal—to act in honor of her own life by preserving Nancy's. To share the affirmation of the value of life that this interaction implies, in different ways, to each, brings the ethical aspects of the situation into Jane's and Nancy's awareness.

Suppose, when Nancy's peril arose, Jane had not been present, and Nancy saved her own life by grabbing onto a log that came floating by. In doing this, she achieved a vital and fundamental goal. She saved her life. The floating log is, obviously, not an ethical aspect of this situation. Nancy's action is its only ethical aspect. Only those aspects of a situation that arise by virtue of human purposes are ethical aspects of that situation.

To put it another way, the ethical aspects of a situation are determined by what is important in the situation. What is important in any situation is determined by the purposes of the agents who can act in it. That something is important, of necessity, implies that it is important to some person in relation to a purpose. This is not to say that what one ought to do in any situation is simply relative to one's desires. To go from "I want X" to "Therefore it is good (or right) that I do Y" is neither ethical nor rational. Justifiability is radically important to ethical decision making. To be the source of justifiable actions, one's desires must be justifiable in terms of their long-term consequences.[2]

A justification is a description in terms of how an action achieves a purpose—the purpose as formulated in a decision or agreement.

To perform an operation, it is justifiable to use a scalpel in order to make the operation possible. It would not be justifiable to use a syringe, scissors, or forceps without a scalpel. These would not achieve the purpose. They would not make the operation possible.

This refers to technical justification, which is not our topic here. Our topic is ethical justification. **An ethical justification is a description in terms of how an action assists the development or happiness of a human by preserving and enhancing his life.**

It is necessary to justify ethical actions in terms of ethical purposes. It is also necessary to justify ethical purposes. An ethical purpose is justified in the case in which it is foreseeably appropriate to the resources and knowledge that one possesses—the resources and knowledge that are necessary to the accomplishment of the purpose. If the actions necessary to accomplish a purpose are inappropriate, then, of course, this purpose is not justifiable. An ethical purpose is justified if the time and resources necessary to achieve it could not be devoted to more vital and fundamental purposes—it does not require time and effort that could be devoted to pursuing greater values. A justifiable action, then, is an action that will foreseeably accomplish a justifiable purpose.

All things being equal, to catch a ride to a restaurant 10 miles from home, knowing you will have to walk 10 miles back may not be easy to justify rationally. In comparison, walking one mile to a restaurant and one mile back is easy to justify.

To act in a way that will foreseeably undermine one's own life or the life of one's patient is not justifiable. To act in a way that will foreseeably undermine the conditions that make agency possible is not justifiable. To act in a way that will foreseeably strengthen one's own agency or the agency of one's patient is justifiable.

To act in order to bring about a change in one's life or the life of one's patient without knowing what effect the change will have cannot be justified. To act to bring about changes that will foreseeably enhance one's own life or the life of one's patient is justifiable.

If that which one desires, or one's patient desires, would increase the ability to achieve that which is desirable, then this desire is justifiable. If it would decrease one's ability, then it is not.

To act against one's knowledge and awareness when this action will affect the life of one's patient or one's own life cannot be justified. It is justifiable to act only when one knows what one is doing.

When circumstances, resources, knowledge, and ability make one's purpose foreseeably possible to achieve, one's purpose is justifiable. When it is foreseeably impossible, then the action is not justifiable.

To embrace a purpose that includes a number of equally valuable purposes is justifiable. If one purpose excludes a number of equally valuable purposes, it is not justifiable.

Without a motivating desire, nothing is important. Desire, itself, is important. Since desire is important, it must always be subject to reason. Reason is an instrument nature has given us to determine what is important—what is desirable—and the means of achieving it. Reason gives human life all of its glory.

A justification must always be achieved through the exercise of reason. It cannot be achieved through desire alone. Desire has no means of self-defense. Reason—and only reason—has the resources necessary to defend itself—to defend an agent's capacity to desire.

Desires are formulated into purposes. There are three types of purpose that determine the ethical aspects of a situation:

- **A purpose set by an individual agent's desire and decision.**
  Desire motivates an agent's action toward every goal. Desire is the principle basis of every human purpose.
- **A purpose set by the recognition of rights.**
  By recognizing the rights of others, one sets uncoerced cooperation as the principle of purposive interaction.
- **A purpose projected and acted upon among individuals through explicit agreements, promises, etc.**
  This purpose must always be motivated by desire and, ethically, must recognize the rights of everyone involved.

THE ROLE OF BENEVOLENCE

Benevolence is a psychological inclination to do good. The quality of benevolence is the most important ethical quality of any health professional. This quality motivates a nurse to act effectively as the agent of her patient. It generates caring and justice. Caring and justice do not exist without benevolence.

To act on benevolence, a nurse must be able to act with understanding. Understanding between a nurse and her patient depends on an agreement on what is to be understood. This understanding must be held in a meeting of the minds, which is the ethical basis of a professional ethic. If a nurse is to do nothing that will bring about harm and everything possible that will bring about good—if she is to act on benevolence—she must know **why she is doing what she is doing**. To have ethical understanding, it is necessary to gain understanding.

There are two ways to gain understanding, which is the first step of a professional's ethical action.

Trial and Error

Because no two human beings are entirely different, every nurse can feel a certain empathy with the human hopes and fears of all persons. She has the basic resources necessary to learn through experience. She can master ethical action through trial and error.

But this is the slowest possible way. While she is learning in this way, she may make many blunders. She may do many things that eventually will bring about harm. She may fail to do many things that would have brought about much good. She may never learn which principles or guidelines are right for ethical action. She may never master the art of applying these principles well in specific cases. Many ethical agents never do.

Reliable Authority

The only other possibility is for a nurse to learn the requirements of right action from a reliable authority on the subject. This leaves the problem of discovering an authority who is reliable.

Certain authorities advise a health care professional to adopt formalistic principles. These are principles that are to be applied indiscriminately without regard to consequences.

If a professional is to act benevolently, she will be able to justify only those actions that bring about an extreme preponderance of benefit over harm. Actions taken ritualistically without concern for the nature of their effects are not actions that are intended to avoid harm and bring about good. Actions can be taken without a prior and specific process of ethical analysis. However, these actions, properly speaking, do not have an ethical motivation.

Animals without the power of reason never reach the level of the ethical. This is true whether they lack the power of reason by nature or by choice. If the actions they take avoid harm and bring about good, this is by accident, not design.

So, for a professional ethic, authorities who offer formalistic rules are not reliable.

Other authorities would advise a health care professional to hold the convenience of others as her principle of ethical judgment. This principle is, at best, the principle of etiquette. Taken beyond the level of etiquette, it ignores the fact that a health care professional has knowledge and a specific function to perform.

It seems apparent that this is inappropriate if a professional has a specific role. This principle would make it impossible to fill her professional role. She cannot hold the convenience of others as the principle of her professional or ethical judgment.

> **Jake, recovering from open heart surgery, is attached to a number of confining apparatuses. Jake is becoming increasingly agitated from inactivity. His family has asked his nurse not to get him out of bed until they arrive. This would be very pleasant and convenient for both Jake and his family. However, his agitation is causing a fluctuation in his vital signs. Proper nursing practice requires Jake's nurse to set aside convenience as a principle of judgment. All rational, bioethical decision making requires precisely the same thing.**

If the principle of convenience were appropriate, robots would make ideal nurses because robots are specifically designed for convenience. A nurse is not a robot, and there is little reason to leap to the conclusion that the betrayal of her knowledge and the sacrifice of her mind is her best answer to the problem of ethical decision making. Still less is a wild vanity that tells a nurse that she is automatically right in her evaluation of a patient's situation because it is impossible for her to be wrong. In order to practice ethically, a nurse must be able to do good while she avoids doing harm. She must be free to use her judgment in the practice of her profession. In fact, **this exercise of judgment is the first demand of beneficence**. So there is still a need to find an authority who understands the requirements of a practice-based ethic.

THE FINAL AUTHORITY

There is an authority who would advise a health care professional to begin from an objective awareness of what is going on in the health care setting. He would ask the professional to exercise her time and effort in acting to help her patient to achieve a passage from his current state of well-being to a more perfect state. He would advise her to justify her actions on the basis of her professional agreement. He would ask her to remain always capable of justifying her decisions and actions on the basis of a practice-based ethic.

This authority, of course, is the patient.

Definition of a Patient

A patient is one who is forced by his circumstances to be passive. **He is one who is unable to take the actions his survival or self-fulfillment requires.**

The patient provides the nurse's reason for being a nurse. It is the patient who enables a nurse to discover the meaning of her work.

Definition of a Nurse

A nurse is **the agent of a patient, doing for a patient what he would do for himself if he were able**. This relationship is codified in an implicit agreement between nurse and patient. In light of this agreement, there is only one authority to whom a professional can turn for bioethical advice—**her patient**.

Centrality of the Patient

It may well be that someone in the health care system is much more sophisticated and has much more academic knowledge about ethics than her patient. But a patient knows far more about his life than this person does. Every health care professional should ask herself whether a professional ethic exists to serve a patient's life, or whether a patient's life exists to serve a professional's idea of ethics? It is impossible to justify the second alternative. So when health care professionals assume it, they do so by denying their patient's right to independence and they do so without justification.

Dilemma 3-2   Mabel has been diagnosed with cancer of the liver. She is also 4 months pregnant with her first child. She and her husband, Mark, had been trying for a long time to have a child. Mabel's physician tells her that to treat her effectively, he will need to use chemotherapy. The chemotherapy will cause severe defects in the child or perhaps abort the fetus. The physician recommends that treatment begin before the child's due date. He suggests aborting the fetus and starting treatment immediately. He believes that to wait until delivery would be detrimental and perhaps fatal to Mabel. He knows that not to wait until delivery would be detrimental and maybe fatal to the fetus. Mabel insists that she wants to live, and that she wants to delay treatment for the child's sake. Charlene is Mabel's nurse.

In making her decision objectively and contextually, Mabel will have to consider every relevant factor. Suppose she refuses to consider one or more factors:

- She might refuse to recognize the fact that she and the baby cannot both survive chemotherapy.
- She might refuse to consider the reason why she ought to have an abortion and begin treatment.
- She might be unwilling to seek a second opinion and to consider the possibility of an alternative means of treatment, perhaps surgery, as a way to save herself and the baby.

In refusing to consider these factors, Mabel is deceiving herself. She is, in effect, violating the standard of objectivity in reference to herself.

Does the fact that Mabel is lying to herself have any ethical relevance to her nurse in their bioethical context? What influence, if any, should this have on Charlene's choices and actions?

All reason is logical and objective. A person can be said to be reasoning only when he or she takes all relevant factors into consideration and follows every fact to its logical conclusion.

In nursing, a major problem arises when a patient should, but will not, face a relevant truth. It is a problem that arises when a nurse tries to communicate with her patient and fails because her patient is unwilling to communicate with her.

How, in the above case, would it be possible for Charlene to communicate with Mabel? (See discussion of this case in Section 5.)

Any bioethical system that does not make the patient, through the agreement, the final authority in ethical decision making drives a wedge between a nurse and patient. It alienates a nurse from her patient, as well as from her professional role. It compels a nurse and her patient to interact in a situation that is unintelligible in principle.

Patients have a justified understanding of the nature of the health care setting and the role of a nurse. There is an agreement between a patient and his nurse. If a nurse respects her patient's rights, she recognizes the patient as the final authority. If she does not recognize the patient as the final bioethical authority, she violates the patient's rights.

Directly or indirectly, every nurse has patients. Some nurses are engaged in education, the purpose of which is the benefit of patients. Others are engaged in administration. The ultimate purpose of the administrator is the benefit of patients. Still others are engaged in research. Again, their ultimate purpose is the benefit of patients.

All these purposes are concretized in the implicit agreement between nurse and patient. Every ethical decision that a nurse makes as a nurse must hold the patient as its central focus. Otherwise, her action misses its mark.

Patients came before health care professionals. Without patients, there would be no such thing as health care professionals.

Her patient is the natural center of a nurse's activity and concern. Nursing is **defined** in terms of the patient. By becoming the nurse of her patient, this action implies that her patient will be the center of her activity.

A nurse's virtue depends upon her actions being justifiable. Justifiable ethical actions are reasoned actions—actions most perfectly calculated to bring about the best result. If her patient is not the center of her concern, a nurse lacks virtue. She is not functioning effectively as a professional. She will be, in effect, passive in relation to her patient.

In the final analysis, not even the hiring institution can ethically come between a nurse and her patient. Every patient expects benevolence and fidelity from his nurse because the nurse is a fellow human being and, therefore, an ethical agent. Anything that interrupts the passage of trust, benevolence, and fidelity between professional and patient violates the right (to realize his rational expectations) of a patient, and the right (to function as an ethical agent) of a professional. This means that a nurse may sometimes have to make a choice. For instance, a nurse has a legal responsibility to function as the agent of her hiring institution. This very seldom or never creates a problem. However, in the unlikely event that her hiring institution clearly proposes to violate the rights of a patient, a nurse has an ethical (and, very probably, a legal) responsibility not to function as its agent (Wilmot, 1998).

A simple examination of the nature of nursing makes the first step of justifiable ethical action obvious. In order to make a bioethical decision, a health care professional, in performing any specific function, must first refer to her agreement with her patient. In matters pertaining to her professional ethical decision making, the patient is the nurse's final authority.

This brings us to another important decision that health professionals need to make everyday: The decision of how she will prioritize her patient visits.

TRIAGE

A triage situation is generally thought of as the scene of a major fire, an automobile or train wreck, a plane crash, or some other dramatic, emergency situation. With the exception of paramedics and emergency room personnel, few health care professionals normally face situations as tense and confusing as these. Yet, every nurse's shift has elements in common with triage situations. Patients constantly enter and leave the health care setting. The conditions and the needs of patients are constantly changing. A nurse's professional actions are best approached with these triage elements in mind. An efficient nurse must be able to meet the ethical demands of the profession with a consistent mind-set and awareness appropriate to the unpredictable.

Every triage situation, from the most catastrophic to the every-day, calls for ethical balance and proportion. Even in situations that are not so complex or demanding as a catastrophic situation, the health care setting itself is a 'low-key' triage situation. Every time a professional enters the health care setting, some patients, or one patient, will have needs greater than others. A nurse masters the problem of ethical balance and proportion as she learns to locate these patients. The mastery of this art (ethical balance and proportion) can be seen in an analysis of a hypothetical situation.

We can conduct our analysis through a thought experiment:

Suppose that there is a situation in which two people, Barbara and Valerie, each have a stake. Their home is burning down and some of their possessions have been left inside. The possession that Barbara might lose is one she would much rather have than lose. The benefit that Valerie might lose is one whose loss would cause her extreme grief. Imagine further that there is a friend, George, inside the house, who has an opportunity to exercise benevolence and to act beneficently in this situation. George can act to assist only one person, either Valerie or Barbara, but not both.

In and of themselves, neither Barbara nor Valerie is intrinsically more deserving than the other. George faces a dilemma. There is not one individual who is the center of the ethical context. Should he assist Barbara or should he assist Valerie? How can he make the best decision?

There is no doubt that some possessions are more important than others. So all possible possessions can be, in effect, evaluated and numbered by George. He can rate them from 1 to 10 according to their importance: Class 1 possessions are those that are least in importance; class 10 possessions are those that are most important. A class 3 possession will not be prized by the person who holds it as much as a class 8 possession will be prized.

In a triage situation, the benefactor (in our case, George), in effect, analyzes the situation in this way:

First, George asks himself: "If Barbara and Valerie were not two people but only one person, what would be the best thing for me to do?" He knows very well that Barbara and Valerie are not one person. But in this situation, in order for him to make the best decision, he must think of them as if they were. He must act as if they were one person with two possessions. He must rescue the possession that would be the more highly rated by this person.

If George could bring just **one** thing from a burning building, he would bring out Valerie's dog rather than Barbara's wedding dress. He would judge that, if Valerie and Barbara were one person, this person would rate her dog at least an 8, while she would rate her wedding dress perhaps a 3.

Although it is one person's dog and another person's wedding dress, George would still rescue Valerie's dog, for the same reason. He judges Valerie's dog, a living thing, to be an 8 to Valerie; he judges Barbara's wedding dress to be a 3 to Barbara.

He would rescue Valerie's dog because this is what is called for in the (triage) situation.[3] The triage situation is an ethical situation where all the potential beneficiaries become one person. The professional commitment is not to an individual, but to everyone involved taken as one person until the most appropriate beneficiary is discovered.

We have been assuming that there is an equal probability of George's being able to salvage either Valerie's dog or Barbara's dress. We have assumed that the risk to George is equal in both cases. The odds for and against a benefactor's being able to bring about different benefits and the risks involved must also be factored in. If George could easily salvage Barbara's wedding dress, but the probability of his salvaging Valerie's dog was very low and/or the peril to him was very high, then it might be more reasonable for him to salvage Barbara's wedding dress.

In a triage situation, a health care professional must sort out all the possible benefits to everyone involved in the situation—wounded soldiers on a battlefield, people injured in an airline disaster, people trapped in a burning building— regardless of whose benefits they are. She cannot make her decision according to the normal professional/patient agreement. Therefore, she must make it according to the benefits that she can bring about.

If a nurse on a battlefield finds a soldier with a broken leg and a sprained ankle, she will fix the broken leg. If she finds two soldiers, one with a broken leg and one with a sprained ankle, she will attend to the one with the broken leg, for the same reason. This is the most important benefit she can bring about.

After an airline disaster, a nurse might treat the severe bleeding of a person with a broken back before immobilizing him. There is something she can do for his bleeding and little she can do for his back. At the same time, his bleeding presents a greater threat to his life than does his back. If she found two survivors, one with severe bleeding and the other with a broken back, she would attend to the one with the severe bleeding, for the same reason that she would attend to an individual person's bleeding before attending to his back.

According to the triage analysis, a health care professional ought to choose her beneficiary according to:

- The importance of the benefit, its ranking on the scale.
- The probability of her being able to bring about the benefit.
- The risks, if any, she will encounter.

In a triage situation, she ought to regard every possible beneficiary as one person. Then she ought to direct her actions according to the most rational desires of this one person.

She ought to do this in a situation where only one person is involved because, in this situation, this is the greatest benefit she can bring about. This is what the rational desire of her beneficiary calls for her to do.

She ought to do this in a triage situation, where more than one person is involved, because this is what an objective reading of the situation calls for her to do.

The analogy between the triage situation and the professional's everyday circumstances is obvious. So is the reasonableness of analyzing them in the same way. If the benefit to one patient is a 6 and no one can receive—or lose—a benefit of 7 or greater, then the professional ought to attend to this patient. If the benefit to another patient would be rated 7 or greater, and providing the first patient's benefit would interfere with the second patient's benefit, the professional should act for the benefit of the second patient.

When it is possible to benefit everyone, then everyone ought to be benefitted. When this is not possible, then those individuals who can be brought the greatest benefit ought to be the beneficiaries of a nurse's actions.

MUSINGS

That which nurses profess (i.e., that which they agree to) is beneficence. Their education, training, and experience fit them to exercise beneficence in the health care setting. The first ethical demand placed on them is that they recognize the nature, demands, and purposes of the health care setting. If a nurse is to act beneficently, she must know why she is doing what she is doing. This is the first step of her ethical professional action. A nurse cannot act, let alone act beneficently, without this awareness. In order to know why she is doing what she is doing, a nurse **must** exercise judgment. This is the first demand of beneficence.

This implies that it is impossible to function under a professional ethic without recognizing the patient as the center of ethical decision making and, therefore, as the final authority as to what happens to him. This requires the nurse to act as the agent of her patient until such time as he can become his own agent.

The nurse/patient agreement is the court of last resort for justifying professional decisions. The more effectively a nurse meets the ethical agreement, the more real she is as an ethical agent and as a professional. On the other hand, it is possible to fulfill the agreement so ineffectively that she will hardly be a professional or an ethical agent at all.

For purposes of analysis, ethical decision making, and ethical action, a triage situation makes every potential beneficiary one person. In the context of a triage situation, the nurse ought to bring about the greatest benefit. She ought to do this because this is, so to speak, what the rational desire of this one person would want her to do.

NOTES

1.   Some physicians still try to keep their patients alive as long as possible. The value of this is obvious. It makes medicine more interesting and challenging. It makes medicine like a game of golf.

The unjustifiability of this practice is also obvious. The physician's profession is not to make a game of his practice nor is it to serve the abstraction "life." The physician's profession is to serve living persons.

Aristotle (1941) observed that, "We can never say that a person's life was happy until its end. For a person may have been successful and contented his entire life. But if, at his life's end, he dies in misery we would have to say that through this tragedy his was an unhappy life." It is better for a physician to allow the final happiness of a patient's life rather than to intensify a patient's misery.

2.   Long-term is relative to the context. For a dying patient, long-term could be a matter of hours or less.

3.   Suppose there had been three persons living in the home and each one, including Valerie and Barbara, had wedding dresses hanging in the same closet. Triage-type thinking would still bring out the dog. A utilitarian would multiply 3×3, which is 9. Nine is more than 8. Therefore, he would save the wedding dresses and let the dog burn to death.

REFERENCES

Brown, B. (Ed.). (1938). *The wisdom of the Chinese.* Garden City, NY: Doubleday.

Mahler, M. S., Pine, F., & Bergman, A. (1975). *The psychological birth of the human infant.* New York: Basic Books.

McKeon, R. (Ed.). (1941). *The basic words of Aristotle.* New York: Random House.

Tunna, K., & Conner, M. (1993). You are your ethics. *The Canadian Nurse, 89,* 25–26.

van Hooft, S. (1990). Moral education for nursing decisions. *Journal of Advanced Nursing, 15,* 210–215.

Wilmot, S. (1998). Nursing by agreement: A contractarian perspective on nursing ethics. *Advanced Practice Nursing Quarterly, 4*(2), 1–7.

CHAPTER 4

The Professional/Patient Agreement

An agreement is a shared state of awareness on the basis of which interaction occurs.

Imagine two people engaged together in some behavior: They are playing volleyball, carrying a plank, going out to dinner, holding hands at the movies, or taking a rocket to the moon. There are three possible sources of their behavior:

- Their behavior is directed by coercion. One person is forcing another to "interact" or both are being forced by a third person.
- Their behavior is directed by deception. One person is aware of what he or she is doing while the other has been deceived into cooperating or both have been deceived by a third person.
- Neither is forced or deceived. They are acting together by agreement. The terms of their agreement are understood by both.

Only the third source of their interaction, only that which is directed by objective agreement, can be justifiable ethical interaction. Force or deception violates the rights of the person who is forced or deceived. There is no way to justify violating a person's rights. "Rights" is defined as: **The product of an implicit agreement among rational beings, made and held by virtue of their rationality, not to obtain actions or the product of actions from each other except through voluntary consent, objectively gained.** It is the fundamental interpersonal ethical concept.

AGREEMENT—THE FOUNDATION OF ETHICAL INTERACTION

That there is objective and voluntary consent between a health care professional and patient means that there is an agreement between them. Objective and voluntary consent never occurs outside of an agreement. This agreement—this shared state of mind—makes their relationship intelligible and, thereby, governs their interaction. It implies that a patient ought to make no arbitrary demands on a health professional. Arbitrary demands do not arise from a shared state of awareness.

Their agreement requires that a nurse be willing to support her patient in any purposes to which he has a right and which are appropriate to his condition. A failure to do this is a failure to act as the agent of her patient.

Dilemma 4-1　A certain patient is in a persistent vegetative state. There is no predictable chance that he will recover from his condition. Some time in the past, he expressed a wish that he be allowed to die if he were in these circumstances. Do beneficence and respect for his autonomy require that he be kept alive?

It can be argued that:

- He must be allowed to die. The unique individual that he once was no longer exists. The recognition of his right to autonomy includes a recognition of the fact that there is no autonomous being to be kept alive.
- He must be allowed to die on the basis of beneficence. Biological survival in the sense of the preservation of electrochemical processes are in no way whatever the equivalent of a human life. If there were any foreseeable possibility of his attaining even the lowest level of a human life, the demands of beneficence might be entirely different. There is no hope for a worthwhile and human life, and respect for his once human dignity requires that he be allowed to die.

On the other hand:

- He must be kept alive. One possesses life only once and life is precious above everything else. Without life, nothing whatever is of any value. The patient's staying alive is a tribute he pays to himself and to his life. Beneficence demands that he be assisted in staying alive.
- He must be kept alive since no one has a right to terminate the life of an autonomous individual. What the patient was in the past is no longer relevant. His autonomy now is the unique nature of his present existence—even if it

is only these electrochemical processes. Recognition of his present autonomy demands that his life be preserved.

The recognition of a patient's autonomy and the motivation of a nurse's beneficence do not necessarily lead to one exclusive and justifiable decision. This is because the bioethical standards, as we shall see, should not, by themselves, inspire a feeling of perfect confidence in any decision. One can be "certain" of the perfection of one's decision only if one ignores the context and makes formalistic decisions irrelevant to the situation. Whenever one makes a relevant judgment, not having absolute knowledge, one may make an imperfect decision. There is no context in which one has absolute knowledge. This is not a reason to ignore the context. It is, rather, a reason to develop the ability to function within a context, to content oneself with achieving that which is objectively possible and desirable, and to ignore an ethical "perfection" that can only be achieved by discarding professional relevance.

In addition to the ethical realities codified in the nurse/patient agreement, there is another ethical reality with which a nurse, as an individual, ought to be concerned. The supreme individual bioethical reality of a nurse is the agreement that she has made with herself—her agreement that she will take on her professional role.

WHAT CAN A COCONUT TEACH US ABOUT ETHICS?

One day, two inhabitants of a jungle village passed a coconut tree. As they passed, a coconut fell from the tree to the ground. An argument arose between them as to who had a right to possession of the coconut. Finally, in despair, they decided to do what seemed to be the only fair thing to do. They split the coconut in half. Each islander took one half of the coconut. They shook hands. Each departed and went on his way.

Could any arrangement be more perfect than this? Surely, this is the ideal resolution to this dilemma? This is the way ethical decisions ought to be made— (?)—the way ethical interaction ought to take place—(??).

In solving their dilemma, they faced a choice between fairness, which is the obvious principle of choice, and a calm and reasoned dialogue that might have led to a better understanding and a more perfect arrangement given their circumstances. They concentrated their attention and discussion entirely upon the context of the situation—that lovely coconut laying on the ground. They communicated nothing to each other about the context of their personal knowledge, needs, and desires.

When they reached their destinations, one villager scooped the fruit out of his coconut and threw it away. He needed a cup and his only interest in his half was the shell that he could use to hold water. The other villager scooped out the fruit and threw away the shell. His family was hungry and he only wanted the fruit.

Had they communicated and come to an agreement based on mutual understanding, one villager would have had twice the number of cups and the other twice as much fruit. They had served their ethical principle—fairness—perfectly, and their own human needs very badly. So it is, all too often, in the health care setting. The more often actions are based on immediate, unquestioned assumptions, the more often the resulting action fails human welfare. The more time that is devoted to generalized ethical theorizing, the less time there is devoted to valuable human concerns.

Every agreement, to be effective, must be aimed toward a final value to be attained through understanding and interaction. The more important this value and the clearer the perception of it, the more powerful its motivational pull will be. Nurses often complain that they do not have enough time to achieve an understanding of their patients. This may be true. Time is rigid and difficult to stretch. But time does not give understanding. Awareness gives understanding. When one knows what to look for, awareness can easily be stretched.

Imagination and distant memories without attention to the present context serve as windows so dirtied up it is not possible to see outside. The only productive solutions are solutions suggested to awareness by the present reality. If they had lifted their awareness to a higher plane, the villagers would have discovered that understanding what we want is a function of desire. Understanding why we want what we want is a function of reason, and a far better way of understanding.

THE ASPECTS OF FIDELITY

The first virtue of a nurse, as a nurse, is fidelity to her patient. The first virtue of a patient, as a patient, is fidelity to himself.

The classic virtues—wisdom, courage, justice, pride, and integrity—are not disregarded by bioethics. They are implied by the principle of fidelity to the nurse/patient agreement. Every virtue and every value involves fidelity, and without fidelity, nothing holds together. Fidelity is essential to a professional ethic. The traditional ethical systems make fidelity impossible.

The virtue of **wisdom** requires a nurse to counsel and interact with her patient on the basis of a well-grounded knowledge. It calls on her to communicate with her patient. It requires her not to interact with her patient on the basis of unexamined beliefs, uncontrolled emotions, self-righteous rationalizations, or an unrealistic opinion of her ethical hunches.

The virtue of **courage** calls on a nurse to defend her own rights and never to violate the rights of her patient. It requires her to accept her own humanity and the humanity of her patient. It requires her to accept the uniqueness and the independence of the patient whose agent she is. Courage is that which inspires independent action for the benefit of a patient. It is shown in her acceptance of a patient's desire even when this desire is not in line with social mores and customs (McFadden, 1996). "If [a nurse] chooses for her patient, she chooses for her profession. . . . This decision requires a certain kind of courage—a courage that . . . is indispensable to the development of a great nurse" (Husted & Husted, 1998, p. 53).

In a bioethical context, **integrity** is a synonym for fidelity.

Pride, as a virtue, inspires a nurse's commitment to herself to strive for professional excellence—to exercise fidelity toward her patient. Pride becomes a virtue when it motivates a nurse, through an agreement she has made with herself, to do nothing of which she need be ashamed, whatever others might think or do (Husted & Husted, 1999). It arises from the expectation she has of herself that she will not fail to act on her professional agreement, and do this as efficiently—as beneficently—as she can.

Very few health care professionals, as patients, would want to be cared for by someone who took no pride in herself as a professional. If one would not want this for herself, it follows that she ought not offer it to her patients.

The virtue of **justice** calls on a professional and patient to exchange values—to take meaning from, and give meaning to, their relationship. This makes justice, in a health care context, a type of friendship.

> To be a friend one must know how to suspend voluntarily his own perspective with its attendant needs and interests; he must know how to discover the principle that is the innermost being of the other; he must know how to use this principle to explore the personal world of the other; he must possess the discretion to will his friend's fulfillment without abrogating his friend's self-responsibility; and he must himself be capable of profound self-disclosure. . . . The will to friendship expresses the recognition that one is in oneself not the totality of goodness but rather an aspect—an aspect that in its actualization summons complementary aspects, willing their actualization together with its own (Norton, 1976, p. 304).

In the context of professional nursing, the "principle" that Norton speaks of, "the principle that is the innermost being of the other," is a patient's fidelity to his health, well-being, and happiness.

In the matter of the villagers and the coconut, the principle was the needs and desires of each villager. By failing to "suspend voluntarily his own [narrow] perspective with its attendant needs and interests . . . to explore the personal world of the other . . . " each, in being fair to himself and to the other, committed an **unseen** injustice against himself and the other.

The function of a professional ethic is to move the implicit professional/patient agreement from a necessary formality to a state of mutual trust—as would befit a state of friendship. A professional "wills her patient's fulfillment without abrogating his self-responsibility." A patient appropriately responds with some level of gratitude. Gratitude is an incentive to friendship. Friendship is an incentive to achieve understanding, concern, and support. A professional appropriately acts with concern. Without this motivation, one cannot act as a professional. Without concern, one cannot be, in its true sense, a professional. Gratitude is the most reasonable response to friendship and concern. Gratitude is a form of justice and, for nurse and patient alike, the most luxurious of the virtues. A patient's freely given gratitude is health care's Olympic gold medal.

The lack of the aspects of fidelity can be seen in the following case.

Dilemma 4-2   Carl has been returned to his room following surgery. The surgery was uneventful and Carl did well in the recovery room. However, he is beginning to experience some pain and asks the nurse for some pain medication. The resident had ordered vicodin 500 mg. About 5 minutes after giving the drug, the nurse came into Carl's room, looking pale, and asked Carl what happens to him when he takes codeine. (It was listed on his chart that he was allergic to codeine.) The nurse noticeably relaxed when Carl replied that he got severe headaches. She then explained that a pharmacist had called and said that vicodin has the same chemical composition as codeine. She said that the resident was at the nurse's station and she would request a new order. The resident resented the pharmacist's interference. He claimed that he knew that vicodin does not have the same chemical make-up as codeine and refused to change the order. What should the pharmacist and the nurse do?

COMMUNICATION

The Biblical story of the Tower of Babel illustrates both the desirability of communication and agreement to the success of interactions, as well as their necessity.

At one time, there was one universal language. A group of Babylonians, discontent with the way God was managing human affairs, decided to build a tower up to heaven, throw Him out, and run things the way they ought to be run. When God observed this waste of time, He became perturbed, and yet He took pity on them.

In order to frustrate the interactions of the builders of the Tower of Babel, God changed the language of each, creating a multitude of languages. This made it impossible for them to communicate, agree, and interact with each other. Work on the tower stopped and eventually it collapsed (Gen 11:1-9).

The Bible asks this question: "How can two walk together lest they agree?" (Amos 3:3). If you think about this, you will see that two cannot walk **together** without an agreement.

Builders cannot build a tower and two cannot walk together without communication and agreement between them. Two cannot interact to enhance each other's lives and overcome conflict when it arises without an agreement. The more closely this agreement is woven into the present context, the more effective the resulting interaction can be expected to be.

An unspoken but formal agreement is absolutely necessary between a health care professional and a patient. Health care would not be an intelligible activity without it. No more than walking together is an intelligible activity if people cannot or do not agree. If an activity is not intelligible, if people cannot understand what they are doing, the activity is impossible.

If people cannot understand what they are doing and why they are doing it, an ethically well-ordered health care system is impossible.

MOTIVATIONS

A most intimate ethical relationship emerges between a nurse and a patient. This relationship is formed on the side of the patient by the desire to regain a state of agency. The loss of agency is a frightening experience. It can involve, to a degree, the loss of the patient's self-image. It can be a very painful experience. It makes a patient dependent on others.

On a nurse's side, the relationship is formed by her response to the patient. Ideally, it will not be formed by any value of the patient's dependency on her, but by her emotional intolerance of her patient's misfortune. This is the attitude that leads most into a health care career.

At the same time, it is to be hoped that a nurse will be strong enough not to wallow in her emotions and allow them to inhibit her actions. She must not allow herself to be "burned-out" by her emotions. And she must not allow herself to resent her patient for being disabled. It would not do for both of them to be disabled.

But not every relationship between nurse and patient is structured in this way. The motivations of each are often deflected from their appropriate course. He may handle his loss of agency and self-image—his state of dependence—in a way that a nurse finds burdensome. Her response to her patient may be resentment. She may be motivated by an emotional intolerance, not of her patient's misfortune, but of her patient himself.

When this occurs, it arises from the breaking of an agreement—an agreement a professional originally made with herself—when she began her career in health care.

A well-ordered nurse/patient relationship involves implied expectations and obligations accepted and agreed to by each. In every case, the expectations and obligations arise somewhat differently. These differences are determined by a number of contextual factors. Chief among these are the condition of the patient and the way in which the ethical character-structures of nurse and patient mesh or fail to mesh in their relationship. Their relationship sets the parameters of their interaction.

The motivating power of a firm agreement is well illustrated in the most famous ethical Biblical parable in the Western world—the story of Solomon and two mothers. King Solomon is, proverbially, thought of as the wisest man who ever lived. He was the king of Israel and served as judge in all disputes between the citizens of Israel.

One night, two women who shared a house bore babies. The child of one woman died, the child of the other survived. When the mother who bore the living child slept, the other woman stole the living child and gave the mother her dead child. Needless to say, a conflict arose between the two women. They were brought before King Solomon.

When Solomon heard the case, he ordered that a sword be brought to him and commanded one of his guards to cut the child in half, giving each woman one half of the child. The woman whose child had died quickly agreed to this arrangement, but the living child's mother instantly asked that the child be given to the other woman (1 Kings 3:16-28).

Solomon made his famous decision on the basis of the nature of an ethical agreement. Solomon knew that the agreement between a woman and a child that is not her own is not so strong, but that she might, out of envy and spite, agree to the death of the child. On the other hand, the agreement between a woman and a child that is her own would never permit her to agree to the death of her child in order to satisfy her resentment.

Solomon's task was to achieve awareness of the true mother's identity. He was able to do this by discovering the power of the contextual interweaving that motivates an agreement.

IS THERE A NURSE/PATIENT AGREEMENT?

The question arises as to whether the professional/patient relationship is based on an actual agreement. For a moment, let us entertain the idea that there is no form of agreement between them. A nurse is motivated to be a nurse. A patient is motivated to be a patient. But their motivations produce no agreement. This is impossible to conceive. Their understanding of their common purpose—to interact—is, in itself, an agreement. If there is no form of agreement between them, there can be no fidelity between them. There is no fidelity between two people who pass each other on the street simply because there is no common purpose between them. Consequently, there is no motivation to form an agreement. A common purpose produces an agreement on the realization of a desired state of affairs. No agreement on a common purpose is possible where there is no common purpose.

Fidelity is made specific by the terms of an agreement. Without the terms of an agreement:

- There is nothing to establish the parameters of fidelity.
- A nurse would have no basis for a stable commitment to her patient.
- A patient has no objective reason to feel confident under a nurse's care.

Without an agreement between them, professional and patient would have no explicit understanding of their roles. Professional and patient could not begin to understand their functioning in the relationship unless an agreement existed between them.

To the extent that there is no explicit understanding of the nurse/patient roles, there is no foundation for their interaction. There is no way for them to structure their interaction. What action could a nurse take if she had no idea what the response of a patient would be? What actions could a patient expect a nurse to take if he had no certain knowledge that she was acting in her capacity as his nurse?

Without a prior agreement, a nurse could not be certain that her patient regarded himself as her patient. Without this agreement, a patient could not be sure that the nurse regarded herself as his nurse.

But these problems do not arise between professional and patient. These problems do not arise, simply, because there **is** an agreement between them. They do not think about it in these terms—and they do not have to think about it—because their agreement solves these problems before they arise.

This agreement makes it possible for each to function. It also makes it necessary for each to apply ethical reasoning to his or her actions. Their agreement is the beginning and the principle of ethical reasoning.

HOW IS THIS AGREEMENT FORMED?

A health care professional does not sit on the patient's bed with pen and paper and say "Now we have to form our agreement." But there is an agreement there nonetheless.

A health care professional walks into a patient's room, where the patient is lying in a bed. Right there, the agreement is set up: "You are my patient. I will be your nurse." "You are my nurse. I will be your patient."

The ethical aspects of the agreement are implied by this. "You are my patient. I will support your virtues—the strength of your character." "You are my nurse. My virtues will interact with yours." Their discovery of each other is sufficient to produce the agreement. They immediately recognize the facts that have brought them together. The agreement arises when a nurse, in effect, accepts a patient's invitation to be his nurse and a patient accepts a nurse's offer to be his nurse.

It is formed by the expectations and commitments of each. Each agrees to satisfy the reasonable expectations of the other. Both agree to live up to their commitment to the other. The nurse is a professional. The patient is an amateur, therefore, the nurse's agreement is necessarily stronger. It ought to be, in Aristotle's words, "fixed and stable" (McKeon, 1941).

Their expectations and commitments establish the agreement between a professional and her patient. This agreement formulates the expectations and the commitments of each. It establishes the boundaries of the successful and unsuccessful in ethical interaction.

It establishes what each has a right to expect from the other—within their interactions. To live up to the agreement is right. To fail to live up to the agreement cannot, in any objective sense, be right. It defines the wrong.

Interactions are complementary actions—actions and reactions—arising between agents on the basis of an agreement. No interaction is possible without an agreement. No interaction between people is possible until they agree upon what each is going to do.

There is no question as to whether an agreement can exist or ought to exist. Without an agreement, professional interaction could not begin.

THE ETHICAL CATEGORIES

A category is defined as, "A specifically defined division in a system of classification" (American Heritage College Dictionary, 1997). The natural categories of ethical action are that it shall be:

- The right thing,
- At the right time,
- For the right reason,
- To the right extent,
- For the right person, and
- In the right way.
  (The ethical categories are not found in Aristotle's book, *The Categories*, but they are discussed in *The Nichomachean Ethics*.)

Under most circumstances, it is impossible to attain perfect certainty. However, in order to justify her decisions and actions, a nurse must attain at least one level of certainty. She must attain the certainty that her decisions and actions have **relevance** to her patient's situation. To deal with the choices she must make, a nurse must develop a sensitivity to what is happening, and she must allow herself to discover that the ideas that pass through her mind are not automatically and infallibly correct: " . . . any ethical analysis that does not take account of uncertainty will be inadequate to the concrete realities of clinical practice" (Beresford, 1991, p. 9).

Every bioethical code obsesses about the right thing to do. This is important, but much more is possible. Through a practice-based ethic, the right thing can be done:

- At the right time—when it is known to be the right thing, and when the action will be most effective.
- For the right reason—with the knowledge of why this is the right thing to do.
- To the right extent—with the appropriate expenditure of time and effort— neither deficiently nor excessively.
- With the right person, when the person with whom one is interacting is the person one ought to be interacting with in relation to whom ethical actions can be known to be relevant and appropriate.
- In the right way—knowing that, not only is it the right thing to do, but that it is being done in a way designed to produce the greatest possible benefit.

A practice-based ethic is different in this: It does not assume that knowledge of the right thing to do is possible without the supporting knowledge of the other categories. Without this knowledge of when, with whom, why, how, and how far action is to be taken, the right thing to do is isolated, out of context, and uncertain. It is this knowledge, if you think about it closely, that forms knowledge of the right thing to do.

AGREEMENT, THE CATEGORIES, AND JUSTIFICATION

If you have a patient, then you have an agreement with your patient. The agreement will enable you to fix your attention on what is relevant. This is what makes him your patient. This agreement specifies what you ought to do. If you keep the agreement, then as easy as flipping a coin, you act to do all of these things—all woven together.

1. What is the right thing to do?
The right thing to do is what you have agreed to do. Otherwise you have agreed to do the wrong thing, which is absurd. What you have agreed to do is your responsibility. The responsibility to do what we have agreed to do is the

strongest obligation we can possibly have. It is the only responsibility we have. The right thing to do is the thing that we have agreed to do. This is our self-evident justification.

2.   What is the right time to take ethical action?

The right time is when action is relevant, and it is relevant when the agreement is in force. If it were not relevant, the agreement would not be in force. This is our only way of knowing—when we ought to take action. The existence of the agreement justifies the timing of action.

3.   What is the right reason for taking ethical actions?

The reason is that one is a health care professional who has agreed to take these actions. Being a health care professional, acting as the agent of a patient is doing for the patient what the patient would do for himself if he were able. This defines your profession. This is your reason to take ethical action. It is a perfect justification for ethical action.

4.   What is the right extent of ethical action?

The right extent is the extent your agreement calls for given the context—the extent implied by your agreement insofar as you agreement is structured by your patient's needs. The agreement is your justification—it is the reason for action. It is the driving force, the "nerve" of what you are doing.

5.   Who is the right person?

The right person is your patient. Who you are as a health care professional is defined in terms of your patient. As a health care professional, your first responsibility is to your patient—to do what you have agreed to do. And your professional agreement is with your patient. This is the reason-for-being of your profession.

6.   What is the right way to take ethical action?

The right way to take ethical action is through actions appropriate to your agreement and the patient with whom you have an agreement.

The right way is shaped by that which is implicit behind the agreement. The right way is the way appropriate to our reading of the character-structures of our patient. Our agreement is based on the objective standards that are behind, and implicit in, the agreement. These structure the nature and needs of our patient and, therefore, the proper forms of ethical interaction. When we are going to do for our patient what he would do for himself if he were able, we ought to do it in the way the patient would—**given the patient's character-structures**.

These are implicit in the agreement. But, we cannot read them in the agreement. Is a patient frightened or not? We cannot read this from the agreement. We can from the patient's actions and reactions.

Dilemma 4-3   Don, a 65-year-old known alcoholic, is admitted to the intensive care unit of a tertiary care hospital with renal complications. He is semicomatose and is unable to communicate or give indication of his wishes. He has been noncompliant with his physician's medical directives for years, has lost his job, his wife, and his children have no communication with him. He currently lives in a one-room apartment over a bar. His mother and sister visit the intensive care unit and communicate with the physicians regarding his care. He does not have a living will and his family indicates that he has never communicated his wishes regarding medical care. The physician plans aggressive treatment of the kidney problem and believes that the patient has a 10 to 20% chance of returning to his prior level of functioning and lifestyle posttreatment.

The elderly mother and the patient's sister communicate to the physician that they want no aggressive treatment for him. They refuse to authorize intravenous antibiotic therapy for the kidney problem; without this treatment, the patient will most likely worsen and die. What should be done?

AVOIDING SMALL MISTAKES

Thomas Aquinas never tired of saying, "A small mistake in the beginning makes for a large mistake at the end." So it is in ethics. It is a mistake to attempt to resolve complex dilemmas by means of hunches, rules of thumb, or any other easy or convenient method. It is no less a mistake to attempt to resolve simple dilemmas in this way.

To tell a patient the truth or not cannot be dealt with on the basis of moral rules. It might be impossible to objectively justify telling a heart attack victim that his wife has been killed. Issues of confidentiality and promise keeping cannot be decided by urges or fixed ideas.

- A psychiatric patient tells a nurse he plans to harm someone. She has pledged confidentiality. Is she bound by this pledge?
- In restraining a senile patient is a nurse practicing unjustifiable paternalism?
- A physician orders a potentially lethal dose of digoxin. A nurse notices this. She cannot contact the physician. Rather than not giving the drug, the nurse gives the normal dose. Should one "blow the whistle" on the physician? On the nurse? On both? On neither?

Unanalyzed rules or guidelines can lead health care professionals into very unjustifiable actions. Ignoring human individuals and the specific realities of their circumstances produces thousands of individual tragedies every day. It is never desirable that the health care system produce more of the same.

Nursing is an interpersonal art. A nurse never acts strictly alone and for herself. Right action demands that she respect her patient's viewpoint. She must be able to tolerate ethical outlooks that differ from her own. Her patient's viewpoint must outweigh the rules she is accustomed to or her own ethical hunches. Someone who cannot accept these limitations on her actions cannot function as a nurse.

Bioethics is, or one day may become, one of the life sciences. For this to come about, bioethics must be optimally appropriate to living and thinking beings (Bourke, 1983). This cannot be done without clarifying and strengthening the health care professional/patient agreement.

Two trends illustrate the importance of agreements: (a) The practice of asking persons to serve as subjects of medical research, and (b) the growing threat of medical malpractice lawsuits.

The Influence of Research

People often serve in medical research. The possibility of exploitation and harm is greater here than in any other aspect of biomedicine. Children, for example, participate in research from which they may gain no benefit. This places an intense ethical responsibility on researchers.

Organ transplants are now commonplace. The techniques of cloning and genetic engineering are being perfected. The application of modern medical knowledge and technology gives rise to the most difficult ethical dilemmas in human experience. Everyone who participates faces these dilemmas.

In general, the role of people engaged in research demands acute awareness of ethical parameters. The application of complex technologies to patients is often hard to justify ethically. Many times, this knowledge and technology complicate otherwise ordinary health care contexts. This calls for very abstract and complex processes of ethical analysis. It is impossible to deal with these issues ethically without rigorous and honest analysis.

The Influence of Medical Malpractice Suits

Nurses sometimes encounter difficulties because of a small mistake. Some are mistaken technical judgments—giving too much or too little of a medication, allowing a large air bubble to be in an intravenous, or harm caused through a failure to notice obvious symptoms. Others involve inappropriate ethical judgments. Today's ethical problems may become tomorrow's legal problems. These problems do not involve mistaken interpretations of the law.

We live in a secular and pluralistic society. In such a society, everything from maximizing the value of interpersonal relations to legal self-defense is achieved through building bridges of ethical understanding between people who are from diverse backgrounds and have different histories. These bridges are made possible by a practice-based moral code.

> If one attempts to chart the conceptual and value commitments of individuals in approaching and resolving biomedical problems . . . one will find a world view that is secular, though not anti-religious . . . the peaceable context of a neutral secular understanding provides the circumstance, within which religious views and special secular traditions can be embraced and pursued in security. A general secular bio-ethics must function as the logic of a pluralism, as the means for the peaceable negotiation of moral intuitions.
>
> Secular bioethics as the provision of a neutral framework to address moral problems in biomedicine is a peaceable solution to the problems of delivery of health care, when physicians, nurses, patients, and individuals generally hold a diversity of moral views. If one is not to . . . impose by force or coercion . . . a particular secular tradition, then one will need to content oneself with a general moral framework that lacks such moorings (Englehardt, 1986, pp. 11–12).

Without bridges of ethical trust between nurse and patient, a nurse may be confronted by an attorney. Attorneys are skilled, professional adversaries whose interests will lie in invalidating a nurse's reasoning and the decisions that result from this reasoning. To attempt to defend herself through a study of the law would be a severely disoriented endeavor for a nurse. Then again, she needs more than a "the-way-I-was-brought-up" defense in order to defend herself. She may have to justify her decisions and actions to a jury of 12 men and women from very diverse backgrounds. Platitudes of duty or ethical intuition or idealistic political inspiration may well prove an inadequate defense.

Ethical decisions are sometimes made from a predetermined ethical commitment. These out-of-context decisions can lead a health care professional into conflict with patients, peers, and the legal system. Medical malpractice suits have made it obvious that unexamined ethical assumptions may not justify ethical decisions. Ethical realities in the specific context must be consciously examined.

A nurse may need an attorney for her legal defense. But she has a responsibility—to herself and her attorney—to know the ethical implications of her actions. This responsibility is entirely her own.

One beneficial result has come from malpractice lawsuits. It has turned the ethical code of health care professionals back to the biomedical contexts in which their decisions are made (Zaner, 1988). This return to reality may prove to be one of medicine's most significant contributions to ethics. It might provide an example contributing to human happiness in general.

JUSTIFICATION, PURPOSE, AND THE CONTEXT

It is logically impossible for a nurse to be able to justify her thinking and yet be blameworthy for her actions. If she has done the best she can, given the context of her knowledge, this is all that can be asked of her.

It is also impossible for a nurse to be praiseworthy for her actions while she is unable to justify the thinking that produced those actions. If the good results that came from her actions were accidental, there is nothing in this for which she can be praised. Both intention and effect are relevant to the quality of an ethical action.

A nurse justifies her actions by describing how these actions would, **foreseeably**, accomplish an ethical purpose. The purpose that justifies her actions is the subject of the agreement. Along with the purpose, there may also be an agreement on the actions that may or may not be taken.

For a decision or action to be justified, four conditions are necessary:

1. The goal of the decision or action must be this predetermined purpose.
2. There must be reason to believe that this decision or action will tend to bring about the accomplishment of its purpose.
3. It must not be an action prohibited by the agreement.
4. It must not be an action that would interfere with actions specified in the agreement.

In a health care setting, the bioethical agreement is an instrument by which both professional and patient can maximize the benefits of their relationship.

Without the agreement, there would be no professional criteria on which to base ethical judgments. Each party to the agreement has ethical responsibilities according to the terms of the agreement, and only according to these terms.

The nature and terms of the agreement between nurse and patient are usually not made explicit for the participants. However, the terms of this agreement are generally known and accepted.

> **A surgical group was consulted to see a patient with an ascending thoracic aneurysm. One of the older surgeons in the group went to see the patient. As the surgeon was very pleasant and informative, the patient and the family immediately built a rapport with her. Because she was so helpful and inspired such a feeling of trust, the patient and family believed that they could trust her and asked her to perform the surgery. The surgeon agreed. The patient's nurse was very surprised to hear that this particular surgeon was performing the surgery. She knew that this surgeon was semiretired and had not done this type of complicated surgery for many years. Should she give the patient and family this information?**

A LOSS OF DIRECTION

Actions that are outside of the nurse/patient agreement often fail to enhance the ethical interrelationship between nurse and patient. They often bring discord into that relationship.

Marie, a nurse at County General, frequently experiences ethical conflict in her interactions with her patients. Sometimes she allows her patient to talk her into negotiating personal problems with the patient's family. Other times, when her patient does not give her the information she needs to care for him adequately, she fails to insist that he be candid with her. There are times when she allows a patient to act toward her with controlling behavior and treat her as if she were a servant. She may allow a patient to hold her responsible for his health while he refuses to cooperate in his regimen of care. Sometimes she reacts to patients in a callous and indifferent manner.

All these activities are outside of the nurse/patient agreement. Sometimes Marie submits to performing them. Sometimes she volunteers.

When these activities are allowed to blur the outlines of the nurse/patient context, they undermine the interaction between Marie and her patients. When Marie neglects her role as professional, her ethical interaction with her patient deteriorates.

Sometimes Marie makes unreasonable demands on her patients. She may lay her personal problems on him or she may take the emotional effects of a bad day out on him. She may decide to place the desires of someone else above her patient's desire.

These practices replace the nurse/patient agreement as Marie's guide to ethical interactions. As the nurse/patient agreement loses its power to direct Marie's interactions, her ethical relationship with her patient comes apart.

In any kind of relationship, all interactions that can be understood and described are formed by an agreement. When it becomes evident that the protection afforded by the agreement is lost, the relationship suffers. One or another party to the agreement feels bewildered and betrayed. He or she may not know why.

The agreement between nurse and patient is an implicit agreement formed by mutual expectations. Being an implicit agreement, it must be protected. Sometimes, even through apparently good intentions, it can be undermined.

Interactions outside of the nurse/patient agreement may have a detrimental effect on a patient's recovery and long-term well-being. They are primary contributors to nurse burn-out. By engaging in interactions outside of the nurse/patient agreement, Marie and her patient lose a clear awareness of what nursing is all about. This awareness is a significant value. Its loss is a significant loss.

PURPOSES AND "PRACTICAL REASON"

Ethical realities are common experiences for all persons. They are not something accepted by mere convention. Nor are they something brought into being by legislation. Everyone has desires and purposes. Everyone must act to achieve his desires and purposes. Everyone faces the need to think before he or she takes actions. These factors cannot exist without bringing the need for ethical thought—for "practical reason"—into existence.

That purpose and value are ethical phenomena pertaining to all people, that all people possess rights, and that all people possess ethical agency are not matters on which one decides. They are ethical realities always already there for one to discover. Ethical realities are human realities, not because people have the power to choose them, but because they are part of human nature and part of the human situation. The supreme interpersonal reality is the network of agreements that makes human interaction possible.

THE AGREEMENT ONE HAS WITH ONESELF

Every nurse ought to examine her life at least to the point where she comes to an agreement with herself that she will be a nurse. To the extent that a nurse has not made this agreement with herself—a commitment to be a nurse—she resembles a patient more than she resembles what she would be if she were a nurse.

> . . . a nurse who directs her long-term actions guided by her awareness of what is needed in order for her to keep that agreement, embraces her profession. A nurse who is inspired by it, and who is dedicated to it, is far less likely to experience burn-out. She experiences joy in taking action. She experiences joy in her ability to take actions—and pride and confidence in acting as she does.
>
> . . . a nurse [who] tries to avoid taking those long-term actions that constitute her professional life breaks the agreement she made with herself to be a professional. She becomes indifferent. She undermines herself as a professional and as a person. If she has replaced her confidence and pride with indifference, she has done this because she abandoned **herself** when she abandoned her profession.
>
> If one is a nurse and is likely to continue to be a nurse, one ought to take the actions the health care professions call for. At worst, this will make life far less boring. At best, it may restore one to the confident expectations and the pride that she began with at the beginning of her career.
>
> Dedication to what one professes—acting on that which one affirms and believes—is sometimes difficult to do. Adversities and frustrations arise. And these attack one's desire and one's sense of self. (Husted & Husted, 1999, p. 17)

But overcoming them through dedication produces pride in oneself as a professional. A patient could not reasonably ask for more and should not find less.

An objective agreement is any agreement in which both parties to the agreement are aware of the reason for the agreement, the terms of the agreement, and the intentions of the other party to the agreement. A nonobjective agreement is any agreement in which one or both parties lack awareness, either of the reason for the agreement, or the terms of the agreement, or the intentions of the other party to the agreement. A nonobjective agreement is a splintered, ineffective agreement. If it is a professional agreement, it will, predictably, fail the responsibilities of the profession.

It is the bioethical standards that make an agreement objective. They are preconditions of an objective agreement. It is important to understand how they function in the interaction between nurse/patient.

Because objective agreement is an essential first step of the nurse/patient interaction, certain standards must be in place. These standards are implied by the existence of the agreement. They arise with the agreement and, at the same time, form its nature.

MUSINGS

The evolution and traditions of health care have produced certain cultural expectations. These also form a bridge of expectations between professional and patient. When a patient enters the health care system, these expectations form an implicit agreement between them. The terms of the agreement are precisely those expectations as each is aware of them.

The appropriateness of the terms of their agreement depends upon their human nature and, especially, the purpose of their interaction. Through necessity, nurse and patient interact under the terms of an agreement to interact. The terms of their agreement guide their interaction. The agreement is a process in which two conscious beings create a resolution between them that becomes their strategy for action. The agreement is foundational.

Agreement is shown in interaction. When the agreement is objective and sound, nurse and patient benefit. When it is not, one or both suffer through it. When an agreement causes suffering, it is a flawed agreement. When it brings objective benefit, it is a sound agreement.

If the desire behind an agreement is a rational, objective, noncoercive, and non-self-destructive desire, then the agreement is the final "court of appeal" concerning interpersonal actions. The purposes of the patient and the nurse, as a nurse, are codified in the agreement. The ethical status of any decision, choice, or action is a function of the relationship of that decision, choice, or action to these purposes. The agreement, then, is the beginning of a nurse's ethical journey—and its principle. The agreement cannot be formed without the patient. It cannot even be understood without the patient. All ethical understanding arises from this agreement.

Everything begins with the agreement, and this is the logical place to bring analysis back to. Where there is disagreement concerning the terms of the agreement, reference must be had to the bioethical standards. We will now turn to these.

REFERENCES

American heritage college dictionary (3rd ed.). (1997). Boston: Houghton Mifflin.

Beresford, E. B. (1991). Uncertainty and the shaping of medical decision. *Hastings Center Report, 21*(4), 6–11.

Bourke, V. (1983, May). *The teleological and deontological dichotomy.* Paper presented at Duquesne University's First Annual Ethics Conference, Pittsburgh, PA.

Engelhardt, H. T., Jr. (1986). *The foundations of bioethics.* New York: Oxford University Press.

Husted, G. L., & Husted, J. H. (1998). The nurse as cynic—etiology and Rx. *Advanced Practice Nursing Quarterly, 4*(3), 51–53.

Husted, J. H., & Husted, G. L. (1999). Agreement: The origin of ethical action. *Critical Care Nursing, 22*(3), 12–18.

McKeon, R. (Ed.). (1941). *The basic works of Aristotle.* New York: Random House.

McFadden, E. A. (1996). Moral development and reproductive health decisions. *JOGNN, 25,* 507–512.

Norton, D. L. (1976). *Personal destinies: A philosophy of ethical individualism.* Princeton, NJ: Princeton University Press.

Zaner, R. (1988). *Ethics and the clinical encounter.* Englewood Cliffs, NJ: Prentice-Hall.

CHAPTER 5

The Bioethical Standards and Their Role as Preconditions of the Agreement

The bioethical standards—the principles that structure the professional/patient agreement—are:

- Autonomy
- Freedom
- Objectivity
- Self-assertion
- Beneficence
- Fidelity

THE BIOETHICAL STANDARDS AND THE PROFESSIONAL/PATIENT AGREEMENT

The health care system has arisen by virtue of specific human desires and needs. These desires, needs, and purposes determine the role of everyone in the health care system. They determine the nature of the role filled by nurses. They are the need for life, health, and well-being—the human need to escape suffering.

A nurse in a health care setting knows why she is there. A patient knows, or comes to know, why he is there. His nurse also knows why he is there. He is there to regain his power to take actions toward his purposes.

A person's power of agency is his power or capacity to initiate and carry
out actions directed toward goals. It is his sense of control over himself—his
actions and his circumstances—when this can be translated into actual control.
A patient comes into the health care setting in order to overcome a physical or
psychological disability. He is there to regain his power of agency. But no patient
regards agency as his final purpose. His final purpose is the goals toward which
he directs purposeful action. Agency is a value in that it enables an agent to
realize purposes beyond itself. But in the health care setting, agency is a goal in
itself. A patient is in the health care setting so that he will be able to return to
the football field, the concert stage, or the factory floor. He is there in order to
return to his family and to his life.

Both the patient and the nurse understand this. This understanding is the **motive**
of their agreement. It shapes the nature of their agreement.

Given the volitional and rational nature of the parties to the agreement, the
bioethical standards are perfectly appropriate to it.

THE BIOETHICAL STANDARDS AS VIRTUES AND RIGHTS: AUTONOMY

Autonomy as Uniqueness

An autonomous agent is one with a right and the power to take actions according to
personal desire and without obtaining permission. One cannot make an agreement
without being an autonomous agent.

The dictionary defines "autonomy" as independence and self-directedness. By
nature, every human is autonomous. Everyone is, at least potentially, independent
and self-directed. Every individual has a right to independence and self-direction.

If it is an easy matter to affirm this, it is also an easy matter to deny it. It is
a truth that is fashionable today. Tomorrow it may come to be thought of as
unfashionable and, therefore, untrue. This would radically undermine the welfare
of patients. It would be a setback for the ethical quality of biomedical practice.

So we have taken the liberty of redefining the term autonomy in order to make
it an undeniable character-structure.[1] This makes it more useful analytically without
losing its connotations of independence and self-directedness.

**Autonomy, as a bioethical standard, refers to the uniqueness of an individ-
ual person. This uniqueness is the specific nature—the character-structures—of that person.**

It is the unique individual who is independent and self-directed and the fact
that every individual is unique is undeniable. Rational animality is the fundamental
nature of every human. We are all part of the same species—rational animals.

Our ethical nature arises from our identity as members of the species. Everyone of this species, by nature, enjoys an ethical dignity equal to every other.

Autonomy as Ethical Equality

Every human being has an individual right to act on his unique and independent purposes and desires (Kikuchi, 1996). Each human being is unique and no human being is less independent than another. No human being is more independent than another. None has a right to override the purposes and desires of others. No one human being has a right to alienate the self-directedness of another. This is so vital to bioethics that we will subject it to a rigorous analysis—an analysis conducted via introspection.

Reflect back on your self-experience and this is what you will find: You, as a human individual, are an organism that moves about from place to place under your own power. You guide your movements through the power of thought—the ability to reason—and the inescapable need to choose and decide.

The choices you must make are, in many cases, the choices every animal organism must make—survival choices. But there are many choices other animal organisms cannot make—choices made via meanings and reason. Many choices you make are highly individualized—choices you make according to your purposes and the meanings you find in your lived world. The rational-animal nature of a human individual endows every person from birth with a striking potential. A nurse's patients, in all but the most extreme cases, enjoy this potential. So do nurses. This potential is a matchless power for growth and development. Throughout the whole species of humankind, each person is different. Our differences begin to emerge when our development begins. This continues through the accumulation of our experiences and the mental and physical actions we take in relation to these experiences.

Through the flourishing of our potential for development, we become what our nature and choices allow us to become. For each of us, who we become is unique. Throughout our lifetime, this uniqueness becomes more and more a part of us and, as we mature, we become evermore unique and more complex.

This is the experience and history of every human individual. Every person begins life as an individual different from all others. Uniqueness increases throughout maturation and development.

The fact that each member of our species undergoes growth and development implies three facts. These facts are vital to bioethical understanding.

1.   You, and every other person, have a right to growth, development, and the pursuit of a destiny. Given your nature and the nature of all the people around you, it is an absurdity to believe that someone else has a right to determine your

development or destiny or that you have a right to determine the development or destiny of another (Husted & Husted, 1997).

2. No two individuals will develop identically. You will be different from everyone else in the world. You and every other person will develop in your own time and circumstances and according to your own experiences, thoughts, and actions.

3. You have a right to be unique. Given your nature and the nature of all the people around you, there is no ground in reality for a belief that your unique character-structure and ethical status are innately superior or inferior to that of anyone else. The nobility or baseness of your character is determined by the individual choices and decisions you make and adopt as your own.

There is no rational, ethical basis for any person to refuse to accept the fact that another is unique in particular (nonaggressive) ways. There is no justification for you to refuse to accept the unique character structure of another—a patient most especially.

Every individual has a right to grow, develop, and pursue his destiny. This requires thought, decision, and action. Each person has a right to think, decide, and act on his own behalf. That is to say, every person has a right to live his or her own life. There is no possibility of another person having a right to think, decide, and act for you. Nor for you to compel the thoughts, decisions, or actions of another. That is to say, no person has a right to take over the life of another.

Every person has a right to be the unique person he or she is. There is no such thing as a character-structure that gives one person the right to choose and determine who another person shall be or the destiny he shall pursue. This, of course, does not imply that a person has a right to pursue criminal or coercive actions against another without being impeded. In this, as in various other places in this chapter, we are discussing the natural relationship between a health care professional and a patient, which they engage in, in normal circumstances. In every instance where coercion or criminality is involved, the situation is quite different. No one has a right to criminal self-determination. A young child may also lack the right to act through self-determination and independence. But to criminalize a person's being who he is, is, self-evidently, an absurd and atrocious violation of his individual rights.

In the right to be unique and to act from that uniqueness, every individual is the absolute ethical equal of every other. How could it be otherwise?

The Right to Autonomy

For these reasons, we define "autonomy" as **uniqueness**. An individual's right to autonomy is his or her right to be the unique rational being he or she is. This obviously includes the right to take independent and self-directed actions. The right to take independent and self-directed actions is the right to freedom. The right to freedom is derived from the right to autonomy. But then, every bioethical standard is derived from the standard of autonomy. If the standard of autonomy cannot be defended, none can be defended. In the context of the bioethical standards, autonomy is the ultimate standard of the rightness or wrongness of a nurse's ethical decisions. If a nurse is to be able to justify her decisions and actions, it is imperative that she be able to defend her decisions in terms of her patient's autonomy.

Unlike an abstract right to self-determination and independence, this right does not depend upon political fashions. The right to be a unique person is nothing more than the right to be human. For any individual person, the right to be human is, quite simply, the right to exist. Quite often, a person's right to self-determination and independence, which is an implicit part of his right to be what he is, can be rationalized away by others. But a person's right to exist and be who he is ethically cannot be put aside. His right to self-determination and independence arises from his right to be who he is. His right to be who he is implies his right to act as who he is.

The reason why an individual makes an agreement, and the terms of the agreement he or she makes, arise from who he or she is.

Dilemma 5-1   Dee, a social worker, is assigned to Anna, an elderly immigrant lady from Eastern Europe who is suffering from emphysema. She is almost destitute and very proud. She will not accept charity. Dee cannot persuade Anna to accept food stamps and Anna is frequently hungry. What can Dee do?

Autonomy as a Precondition of the Agreement

A nurse and a patient must be different. They do not do the same thing. They interact. It is very fortunate that nature has made everyone unique and different. Otherwise, no agreement—no trade—no interchange of values—between people would be possible.

Autonomy—the uniqueness of every person—is a precondition of the health care professional/patient agreement. It is, itself, an agreement that is implied and assumed in every other agreement. As an agreement, it is a bioethical standard. As an essential precondition of the nurse/patient agreement, it is a bioethical principle. It is the cause of an agent's motivation to action—the motivation that causes every action he takes.

For either professional or patient to violate the autonomy of the other is to act as if no agreement exists between them. For this is, implicitly, to deny a necessary precondition of the existence of an agreement. If no agreement exists, then no stable and intelligible relationship can exist between them. When no stable and intelligible relationship exists, there is no such thing as **nurse/patient** interactions.

As a bioethical standard, respect for autonomy is the necessity placed on health care professionals of accepting the uniqueness of a patient. This is simply accepting a patient. A nurse who does not accept the uniqueness of her patient is performing a perverse form of nursing.

Autonomy, as a patient's right, is his right to be who he is. By right, his desires and actions arise from whom he is.

Recognition of the right to autonomy involves a willingness not to interfere with actions toward goals that are not one's own. It involves recognition of the fact that a patient's purposes cannot be abridged on the grounds that the patient or his purposes are different from some societal norm. A nurse has no right to attempt to frustrate a patient's purposes, no matter how much they differ from or clash with her own. Nor does any health care professional have a right to either enforce or interfere with an obligation that a patient has chosen for himself.

> **Peter has carcinoma of the lung. The attending physician decides that chemotherapy is the treatment of choice. The physician does not consult with Peter. He is convinced that Peter has an obligation to himself to undergo the treatment and, therefore, need not be consulted.**

> Despite efforts to respect autonomy, it is almost impossible to remove a sense of coercion when the patient is weak, helpless, and at the mercy of others. Furthermore . . . physicians are strongly influenced by their personal values and unconscious motivations. . . . (Orlowski & Kanoti, 1986, p. 48)

The notion of an enforced obligation that a patient has to himself is ethically unintelligible. Health care professionals are not, nor ought they be, enforcers of anything. An agent's autonomy is recognized through the recognition of his freedom to decide for himself.

A patient does not make a choice or decision in a vacuum. However, it is the health care professional's responsibility to remove as much coercion or undue influence as possible.

FREEDOM

Freedom as a bioethical standard is self-directedness—an agent's capacity and consequent right to take long-term actions based on the agent's own awareness of the situation in which he acts.

One can possess freedom without making an agreement, but one cannot make an agreement without possessing freedom.

Susan is walking down the street. Suddenly she is struck by the attractiveness of the dresses in a department store window. She stops to admire them. So far, Susan is passive. The dresses are, so to speak, coming out and influencing Susan. Susan is taking no external action in relation to them. In the context of this experience, she is a patient.

Susan decides to buy a dress. She enters the department store and chooses one. She makes an agreement with a clerk. Susan pays the clerk the price of the dress and acquires it. In these experiences, Susan is active. She has become an agent taking action toward a goal.

Susan might very well have decided not to buy a dress. This would also have been an action and an exercise of her freedom. But it would have been an exercise of her freedom, not involving any agreement with any other person. It would have been a **decision** involving only an agreement with herself.

Suppose Susan was unable to decide which dress to buy. Her subsequent actions, including her agreement with the clerk, would never have occurred. She would have been passive throughout the whole event. Throughout this entire event, Susan had the power and right to exercise agency or to refrain from engaging in positive action. Without the power and right to make a voluntary choice, there can be no "meeting of the minds."

Without a meeting of the minds, there can be no agreement. Without agreement, there can be no ethical interaction. Freedom is presupposed in any attempt at ethical interaction.

Dilemma 5-2   Edgar has been in the hospital for almost 12 weeks. His prognosis is very poor, but the family remains insistent on the patient's remaining a full code, despite the physician's opinions on the poor prognosis and his present and future quality of life. Edgar has multiple medical problems, including metastatic cancer. He has been heard to say on a number of occasions, "I do not want to live." He now is semicomatose and cannot make his wants known. The family remains unrealistically optimistic.

When one person refuses to respect the rights of another, a meeting of the minds between them is impossible. The conflict between them leaves no room for an agreement. In the absence of an agreement, there is no basis between them for trust and ethically guided interaction.

THE INTERWEAVING OF AUTONOMY AND FREEDOM

An agent possesses freedom in two senses:

1. In a biological sense, every agent possesses freedom in that he has the potential for taking independent actions.

2. In an ethical sense, every agent possesses freedom since there is nothing in human nature to justify one agent's right to interfere with the independent action of another. Whatever rights an individual possesses, he possesses by virtue of his human nature.

Every ethical agent possesses an identical human nature. Therefore, every ethical agent possesses identical rights. That one human is more human than another and, by this fact, possessed of "superior" rights is an absurdity. It is the same type of absurdity the pigs in George Orwell's *Animal Farm* (1945) were guilty of when they declared that, "Some animals are more equal than others."

All ethical agents possess freedom equal to that of all other ethical agents and nothing more. An agent's existential freedom is enormously increased by his possession of rights. But it is limited by the fact that others also possess rights. No agent has, **ethically**, freedom to violate the rights of others.

Autonomy accrues to a patient by virtue of the fact that he has the power to pursue goals peculiar to his own unique desires. Freedom accrues to a patient by virtue of the fact that reasoning agents can and must plan and take actions directed toward future goals.

An agent's freedom is his right to determine for himself the meaning and importance of a context. It is also freedom to:

- Form purposes,
- Pursue his goals, and
- Bring about changes.

It is freedom to act with practical reason.

One implication of freedom is the doctrine that nothing should be done to a patient without the patient's consent. It is a direct implication of the standard of autonomy. Autonomy permits a patient to be what he is. Freedom permits him to act for that which he perceives as his own benefit. Under the standard of freedom, one may not interfere with a patient's purposes. One may not compel a patient to act, or to submit to the actions of others, against his will.

Freedom is established by the very same line of reasoning as autonomy. To violate the standard of freedom is to violate the nature of an agent. It is particularly incongruous in a biomedical setting. **The whole purpose of a biomedical setting is to enable a patient to regain agency, not to assist him in losing it.** To work for a patient's agency, and, at the same time, to violate it, reveals a "contradiction" in one's actions. There is no such thing as an ethically justifiable contradiction. The agreement does not call for a patient to deliver whatever power of agency he possesses to a health care professional. A person's right to freedom is his right to the privacy of his will.

Suppose someone wrote a biography of Paul McCartney. Someone else wrote a biography of John Lennon. A third biographer wrote about the life of George Harrison, and a fourth, the life of Ringo Starr. Suppose further that each biography discussed the life of its subject without ever mentioning the existence of the other three. These biographies would miss that which was of historic significance in the life of the Beatles. None would be a complete, or even a relevant, account of the life of its subject.

The case is very much the same with autonomy and freedom. Neither can be understood without the other. They are intrinsically intertwined.

That an agent is autonomous, that he possesses desires, values, and purposes peculiar to himself, is the sole reason he requires a right to freedom. It is the reason why rational agents implicitly agree to respect these rights. Otherwise, if an agent did not possess autonomy, his purposes might be best served by his being in a harness.

At the same time, that an agent has a right to freedom means that he has a right to autonomy. Freedom is freedom to be autonomous.

Freedom as a Precondition of the Agreement

Whenever two people reach an agreement, each implicitly assumes that the other possesses freedom—the power and the right to act toward his own goals, guided by his own awareness. This is a necessary precondition, and a principle, of their agreement.

If a nurse remembers the necessary preconditions of an agreement, she has a powerful ethical resource. For, in the very nature of health care, every nurse has an agreement with every patient. Freedom is one of the necessary preconditions of the nurse/patient agreement, as it is of every agreement.

A nurse should never forget that a patient has the right to free decision, choice, and action. To forget that a patient has this right is to forget that there is a nurse/patient agreement. If there was no nurse/patient agreement, there would be no nurse/patient relationship. If there was no nurse/patient relationship, the nurse would have no right to take any action whatever in regard to the patient.

OBJECTIVITY

As an intellectual capacity, objectivity is a person's ability to be aware of things as they are in themselves apart from his awareness and evaluations. As a physical capacity, objectivity is a person's ability to act on this awareness.

As a bioethical standard, objectivity is a patient's need to achieve and sustain the exercise of his objective awareness. In relation to the standard of autonomy, it is a patient's right to be supported in the act of exercising and acting on objective awareness.

It is logically impossible to have confidence in an agreement if one cannot have confidence in the understanding of the people making the agreement. For then, one could not achieve certainty concerning the existence of an agreement. An uncertain agreement—one in which no one has any confidence—is really no agreement at all.

People can understand each other without entering into an agreement. The sun is bright. Paul reports to Marcy that the sun is bright. Paul has brought understanding to Marcy. But no agreement has been entered into between Paul and Marcy.

On the other hand, no one can enter into an agreement unless the parties to the agreement have reached a meeting of the minds. Harry and Bill agree to share the driving on a trip to Fort Lauderdale. Harry does not know how to drive. There cannot be a meeting of the minds. The agreement that Bill assumes to exist really does not exist.

One can achieve objective awareness without entering into an agreement. But one cannot enter into an agreement unless one has achieved objective awareness.

Long ago, people began to communicate with each other on an abstract level. Early on, some genius of our species noted that, if people are going to communicate and interact on this level, objective awareness is of the highest importance. Without an objective awareness established upon objective facts, no person could trust herself or her own judgment. A fortiori, there could not be trust among humans. Without trust, there cannot be communication and interaction.

If people do not communicate with each other objectively, they will suffer through their interaction and communication. Their only recourse will be to give up communication and interaction.

All the bioethical standards, in one way or another, involve objectivity. The standard of objectivity requires that a nurse accept (tell herself) the truth concerning the unique nature of her patient and her patient's inalienable right to direct the course of his life. The standard of freedom implies the need of objective awareness. It also implies an emotional level wherein the ability to act on objective awareness is not undermined.

Dilemma 5-3   Luke is a young man who is dying from a severely debilitating disease. He has been ill for a long time. Betty, a dietician, is called in as a dietary consult by the physician. The physician wants to begin total parenteral nutrition on this patient to prevent further debilitation. Luke is no longer able to communicate his wishes and he has no immediate family to consult. Betty believes that this method of treatment is inappropriate for a person like Luke. Betty discusses this with Luke's nurse, Catlin. What, if anything, should Betty and Catlin do in this situation?

Objectivity as the Precondition of the Agreement

One person cannot make an agreement with another person unless he rightly expects objectivity from that other person. There can be an agreement only where there is a meeting of the minds. Each party to the agreement must have an informed knowledge of its terms. Without this knowledge, a person obviously could not be party to an **agreement**. Each party to an agreement must be certain of the terms of the agreement. He can be certain of the terms of the agreement only if he has an assurance that he has access to its objective terms. Therefore, objectivity is a standard—an ethical measure of an agreement. As a necessary precondition of an agreement, it is a bioethical principle.

SELF-ASSERTION

Self-assertion as a bioethical standard is the power and right of an agent to control his time and effort. It implies a person's self-ownership.

As freedom is the right to pursue courses of action without being interfered with, self-assertion, in its broadest sense, is the right to control one's time and effort—one's right not to be deceived or coerced into action.

One can be a self-assertive person and never make agreements. Making an agreement may involve giving up part of one's control of one's time and effort. But the practical benefits of making agreements would not be possible to one who did not possess this right. Many of the benefits of long-term planning, whether this involves agreements with others, would be lost to a person who could not control his time and effort.

A patient voluntarily gives up a part of his self-control to a health care professional. This much is obvious. There is, however, no reason for a health care professional to assume that her patient gives up all right to self-control.

Self-assertion, as a standard, is the health care professional's obligation to protect her patient from coerced action or undesired interaction. The whole world does not have the right to determine a patient's actions. No one has. This is also implied by the patient's right to freedom. No one has a right to violate a patient's rights. Nor does any health care professional have a right to violate a third person's rights for the benefit of a patient.

A patient's right to self-assertion is one right that a health care professional ought to be especially careful to protect. A violation of this right involves the unsupportable implication that the patient has no human rights. But the worth and dignity of a health care professional rests in the fact that she deals with those who do possess rights and human dignity.

Demeaning the status of the patient involves demeaning the status of the health care professional herself. Protecting the self-assertion of a patient is precisely a recognition of his worth and human dignity. Protecting the worth and dignity of the patient is a professional's tribute to her own worth and dignity. "Personal control and autonomy [freedom] are powerful components in terms of life satisfaction, survival, and how one defines one's role . . . " (Rice, Beck, & Stevenson, 1997, p. 32). There can be no justification for denying this to a patient.

Dilemma 5-4   A patient exercises his self-ownership by bringing himself into a health care setting. He comes into the hospital with a liver condition. While he is in the health care setting, he becomes quite friendly with his nurse. One day, he swears his nurse to secrecy. Then he informs her of a certain fact regarding his condition. During the course of his treatment, the patient becomes incapable of making a decision. This poses a dilemma for his nurse around the standard of self-assertion. She has promised to maintain confidentiality in the matter he related to her. But the information the patient gave her is now needed by the physician to treat him effectively.

Self-Assertion as a Precondition of the Agreement

Individuals must enjoy some degree of self-control and isolation from one another. Without the freedom from distraction provided by this isolation, an individual could not maintain his integrity or function effectively. A patient comes into a health care setting in order to attain, maintain, or regain his integrity and his capacity to function.

Everyone has a need for the power of self-assertion. This requires a certain degree of isolation. This isolation is essential for a person's self-awareness. It is also essential for the exercise of a person's freedom. This isolation—this moral defense against coercion—is the value that the standard of self-assertion offers a patient.

If a person has no right to self-assertion, then there is no such thing as self-ownership. If one has no right to self-ownership, he has no right to make an agreement. One cannot make an agreement for the disposition of that which he does not own. He cannot agree to exert effort if he does not own and control his effort. He cannot agree to devote time if he does not own his time. Only a person who has a secure hold on his time and effort, can exercise the virtue of self-assertion. An agreement could not be formed without the exercise of this virtue. Therefore, it is a principle of agreement.

To make an agreement with one who lacked the power of self-assertion would be as useless as trying to iron a blouse with an ice cube. Every professional must be, at least implicitly, aware of the power of self-assertion in a patient with whom she makes an agreement. She has no right, thereafter, to act as if she lacked this knowledge.

BENEFICENCE[2]

The concept of beneficence refers to the fact that every agent acts to achieve benefits and to avoid harm.

As a bioethical standard, beneficence is the power of an agent, and the necessity he faces, to act to acquire the benefits he desires, and the needs his life requires.

It is a scandal of modern medicine that a professional's ability to exercise beneficence is severely circumscribed.

> In February 1985, [the] New Jersey appellate court ruled that a hospital had the right to dismiss a nurse who refused, for "moral, medical and philosophic" reasons, to administer kidney dialysis treatments to a terminally ill double amputee. . . . Mrs. Warthen [the nurse] asked to be replaced, arguing that she could not submit the man to dialysis because he was dying and the procedure was causing additional complications. She . . . was fired. . . . The three-judge appellate panel agreed with the hospital . . . (Humphry & Wickett, 1986, p. 122)

Mrs. Warthen was motivated to take her position by her understanding of beneficence and objectivity. Most health care professionals would agree that her stand was beneficent—and objective. No doubt the hospital where Mrs. Warthen worked held the value of beneficence in high esteem. But the value of their beneficence was not very influential in this instance.

Health care professionals sometimes appeal to a concern for objectivity (reduced to truth-telling) in order to violate the requirements of beneficence. This is one instance of an apparent conflict between the bioethical standards.

Dilemma 5-5   Sixteen-year-old Robin is dying from lupus erythematosus. She is very fearful. Toward the end, she screams, over and over, "Don't let me die!" Robin's parents are called to the hospital, but before they arrive, Robin dies. They ask Robin's nurse if their daughter's death was peaceful. Robin's nurse dutifully relates all the details of Robin's death. Empathy would have made Robin's nurse weak. For Robin's nurse to share the human feelings of Robin's parents might have made her relating the truth unbearably painful. She is strengthened in her duty by apathy. She finds, in the absence of feeling, a sort of strength. If empathy among persons is a virtue, then this context does not call for truth. But if submission to the duty to tell the truth is a virtue, then empathy is a vice. There is no benevolent purpose served by Robin's parents hearing the truth. The consequences of the nurse's truth-telling are entirely evil.

Beneficence is an intention to assist a patient's efforts in attaining benefits he desires. It is conceivable but not very likely that a person could act beneficently without making agreements. Under most circumstances, it is inconceivable that people without a sense of beneficence would make agreements. What possible purpose could be served by making an agreement with someone who had no intention of helping us to attain a benefit that we desire.

Beneficence is the act of assisting a patient's effort to acquire benefits that he desires. This standard counsels a professional to relate to a patient in a way that will always be maximally beneficial for the patient. It implies that a professional should scrupulously avoid interacting with a patient in any way that might cause unnecessary and avoidable harm.

As to diseases, make a habit of two things—to help, or at least to do no harm. (Hippocrates [460–377 B.C.], *Epidemics*, Book I, Sec. XI)

Beneficence is a quality of actions. It characterizes actions that are motivated by benevolence. Benevolence is a frame of mind. It is a consistent attitude of good will toward another or toward oneself. Beneficence is the practice of acting on the prompting of good will—the desire to benefit one with whom one empathizes.

Patients do not always find beneficence in a health care setting. The situation is far from perfect today, but it is infinitely better than it once was. The conditions during her time led Florence Nightingale (1991) to declare that it is a strange but necessary standard to enunciate as the very first requirement in a hospital that it should do the sick no harm. Beneficence is, of necessity, an integral part of the nurse/patient agreement.

A beneficent nurse acts with empathy for her patient—and without resentment or malice.

Although a patient, on entering a hospital, makes a commitment to let the hospital function as a hospital, a patient or a patient's family has an absolute right to decline treatment or any form of abuse. "To force a patient to undergo treatment against his or her wishes . . . constitutes both a violation of autonomy, and the infliction of harm. In cases such as these, the autonomous patient determines what constitutes unwarranted suffering" (Fowler & Levine-Ariff, 1987, p. 193). Conflicts can arise concerning the demands of beneficence and the natural function of a health care setting. These are, in fact, the most common bioethical dilemmas. But, in the final analysis, none are genuine dilemmas.

Beneficence as a Precondition of the Agreement

Each individual person has a need to achieve good and avoid harm. Beneficence is a bioethical standard (and, more generally, a standard of ethical action) because humans are beings who can impede and injure one another. This is proved by the fact that they do impede and injure one another. They can also agree on and exercise beneficence toward one another. This is proved by the fact that they do exercise beneficence toward one another. The standard of beneficence arises when ethical agents have attained a sufficient degree of rationality to recognize the advantages of "doing good or at least doing no harm" (Hippocrates).

The biomedical sciences are a concrete expression of this beneficence. Beneficence is a precondition and principle of agreement.

FIDELITY[3]

Fidelity, as a bioethical standard, is an individual's faithfulness to his autonomy. For a nurse, fidelity is commitment to the obligation she has accepted in her professional role.

A nurse lives her profession through fidelity. Fidelity is commitment to a promise. This is the promise to honor her agreement with her patient. But a nurse's fidelity is not fidelity to an agreement. It is a commitment to her patient (Husted & Husted, 1995). More precisely, it is fidelity to her patient's life, health, and well-being.

A nurse has an obligation to attend to her patient in the sense of providing care for him. She also has an obligation to attend to him in the sense of listening to him and counseling him. At the very least, she has an obligation to protect him from preventable harm.

Any person, including a nurse, has a right to speak out to protect any other person, including a patient, from harm. This is an aspect of beneficence. When a nurse "blows the whistle" to protect a patient, she relies on something more central to their agreement than mere benevolence. Whistle blowing is an aspect of fidelity.

For a patient, the demands of fidelity are quite different from those for the nurse. This because the roles of nurse and patient are very different. A nurse's role, by definition, is much more active than a patient's.

This certainly does not mean that a patient has no moral obligation to exercise fidelity. If a nurse is to be the agent of a patient, the patient must cooperate in the exercise of this agency. This is an exercise of his responsibility to be faithful to his life. Fidelity to himself and to his nurse is simply a recognition of what a nurse is. This includes the avoidance of behavior that makes contradictory demands on her. For example:

- After surgery, a patient expects a nurse to protect him from pneumonia. But he refuses to cough and practice deep breathing postoperatively.
- A patient expects a physical therapist to help him become more mobile after a stroke. But he refuses to go to physical therapy.
- A patient expects a nurse to protect him from injury. But he refuses to get assistance before getting out of bed.

If a patient does not honor the terms implied by his agreement with his nurse, he violates this agreement. Worse still, he violates his own purposes. If a nurse does not honor the terms implied by her agreement herself, she violates her purposes—she disconnects from her life.

Fidelity always involves an agreement. So, of course, it is not possible to practice fidelity without making agreements. It is also not possible to keep an agreement without practicing fidelity. An agreement made without the anticipation of fidelity is a logical impossibility.

However, in expecting fidelity from her patient, a nurse must always bear in mind the incapacities that his condition forces upon him. When she does not receive the cooperation of a patient, she must remember her commitment to her profession. Even when things cannot be done perfectly, she must do the best she can. This is her obligation to her profession—and to herself.

Dilemma 5-6   Ruth, an 80-year-old, is terminally ill. She has been on the unit for weeks. Family members rarely visit. They have refused to allow the physician to write a do-not-resuscitate order. The nurse, Madeline, sees her patient suffering: Ruth's breathing is labored; she is not fully conscious; yet she is restless and seems to be experiencing some pain. On past admissions, she has told Madeline not to pound on her at the end, just let her go in peace. However, she has not made a Living Will. One day, Madeline comes back from her dinner break and goes in to check on Ruth. She finds that she has stopped breathing. What should Madeline do?

Fidelity as a Precondition of the Agreement

Agreements serve a purpose in human lives. This purpose is the benefit that people gain through cooperation. Through cooperation, ethical agents are able to achieve good and to avoid harm. It contradicts the nature of an agreement, then, that people would form an agreement and, within the confines of that agreement, refuse to do good or at least do no harm to one another.

It is a very easy matter to see that no agreement between two people can be maintained if the standard of fidelity is not maintained. **Fidelity is an outgrowth of the recognition of the other standards.** To gain the benefits of interaction, individuals must be able to rely on each other. This reliance is made possible by the implicit and explicit understandings upon which their interaction is based. Fidelity is fidelity to these understandings. It is an essential principle of agreement. Agreement would not be possible without fidelity.

A denial of the relevance of any of the bioethical standards to the agreement cannot be logically justified. In one way or another, the denial would make a claim that, if it were true, would undermine all possibility of an agreement. To greatly simplify the matter, it is rather like someone declaring, "I don't speak a word of English," where the very fact that this claim is made in English falsifies it.

If a nurse makes an agreement with a patient, she makes an agreement with a being who is autonomous, free . . . and the rest. If she interacts as if he were not autonomous, free, etc., to this extent she violates her agreement. To the extent that she violates her agreement she refuses to act as a nurse. Her agreement and actions contradict each other. This is important. A nurse does not make any ethical agreement after the nurse/patient agreement. Every ethical agreement is implied in this agreement.

AGREEMENT AND CONTEXT

The center of the nurse's ethical context cannot be posterity, the environment, cultural values, or anything but her individual patient. Her professional agreement cannot be with anyone but with her patient. The limits of the ethical context lie entirely within her professional agreement.

Dilemma 5-7   Maria Reyna is a 32-year-old Mexican American female who is being seen in the in-patient mental health center for symptoms of depression, anxiety, and loss of appetite. Maria is first generation in the United States. She is married to Ray and they have a 7-year-old daughter. Ray was born in Mexico, but has lived in the United States for 12 years. Both are bilingual in Spanish and English. Ray told the psychiatric nurse on admission that his wife is experiencing sustos. (*Sustos* is a belief in the Mexican American culture that means loss of soul.) He said that his wife came out of the house 1 week ago to look for their 7-year-old daughter and witnessed a near miss between a van and her daughter playing in the street. Ever since this event, Maria has been experiencing these symptoms, and Ray believes that she will not be well until the soul is reunited with her body. Ray and his family have asked that a *currendera* (folk healer) be called to see his wife in the hospital to perform a healing ritual to reunite the soul with the body.

After the interview with Ray, the nurse met with Maria to discuss her perception of her symptoms. Maria told the nurse that she does not know why she is feeling "so bad," but wants help from professionals. Maria knows that her husband thinks her illness is due to sustos. She does not have the heart to tell him that she does not believe that this is the cause of her condition. Maria stated that, in some cases, she does believe in sustos, but not for her in this case (Zoucha & Husted, 2000, p. 336).

Without the nurse/patient agreement, no bioethical context would ever arise. The nurse and the patient's situation and interactions would be unintelligible. Only in the context of the agreement do they become intelligible. Only through an agreement does a nursing situation become a context.

Nursing, as an activity, has a nature entirely its own. It is different from all other types of activity. It is an activity oriented toward specific purposes. It is characterized by specific interpersonal interactions. The nature of these interactions is determined by the nature of nursing as a science.

Within the interpersonal relationship of nurse and patient there is an interweaving of expectations and commitments. These expectations and commitments shape the nature of the relationship for both nurse and patient.

This complex of expectations and commitments between nurse and patient forms an agreement between them. Each agrees to satisfy, to one extent or another, the expectations of the other. Both agree to live up to the commitments each has made to the other. Their agreement is a recognition by each of the expectations and commitments existing between them.

Interactions between people must be based on expectations and responsibilities that are known by each. The interweaving of their purposes and obligations form the agreement between them. Without this agreement, there would be no pattern to their interactions. Without intelligible patterns of interaction between nurse and patient, nursing would not be a specific activity. It would refer to nothing.

MUSINGS

Whenever an agreement exists between two people, each has expectations and responsibilities as a result of that agreement. This is true of the professional/patient agreement, as it is true of every agreement. It is expectations that motivate a person to take on the responsibilities of an agreement.

Every agreement consists in the specific terms of that agreement and a promise by each party to the agreement that he will be faithful to it. Keeping this promise requires that each be aware of and respect the nature of the other. Without this implicit awareness, there simply is no interaction. Fidelity to one's awareness is basic to agreement and interaction.

Figure 5.1 is meant to be a guide for those using the theory of a Symphonological practice-based ethic. It gives a visual picture of the concepts and their approximate

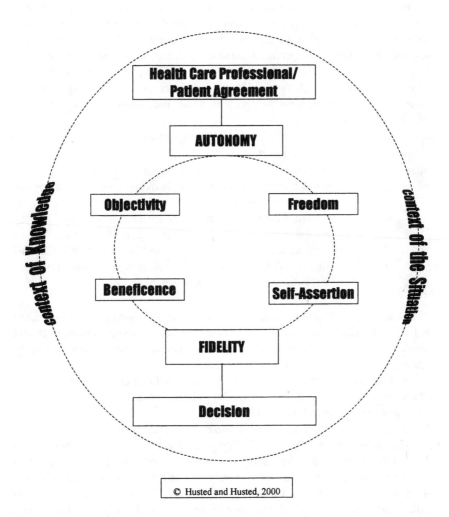

© Husted and Husted, 2000

FIGURE 5.1   Husted's symphonological bioethical decision-making guide.

relationships. However, no diagram can convey the meanings, relationships, and use of the theory without an understanding of the theory itself.

NOTES

1.   Certain terms used in the book are redefined for the sake of maximum usefulness. Autonomy is one of these terms.

The way a person exercises his or her self-governance and right to take independent action is not determined by the mere fact that the person is independent and self-governing. It is determined by that person's unique desires and values—his or her unique character-structure. A nurse understands her patient, or anyone else, better if she makes herself aware of the ways in which he is unique than she does if she simply makes herself aware of his independence and right to self-governance alone. For the technical sense in which terms are used in this text, the reader is referred to the Glossary.

2.   In the first edition, we offered the following dilemma:

Dilemma 5-8   Martha has bone cancer and is suffering excruciating pain. Treatment has been unsuccessful. She is dying. Heroic measures are used in order to keep her alive. A nurse's suggestion that Martha be allowed to die is met with outrage from her colleagues. The only benefit the nurse's colleagues can envision is Martha's sacrifice to "ethical" ideals essentially irrelevant to Martha's situation. If ethical ideals do demand this, it is unfortunate because this idea certainly debases the concept of benevolence.

It is no longer demanded by law that a suffering and dying patient be tortured as long as possible. These ethical ideals are now recognized as unethical. In this situation, the law has caught up to bioethics. Previously, these ideals were merely inhuman. Now, they are both inhuman and illegal.

The question of euthanasia is one of the most difficult questions in bioethics. Often the analysis of a different dilemma will illuminate the way in which less difficult dilemmas ought to be analyzed.

Therefore, we have retained the analysis of this dilemma.

3.   If a patient fails to exercise fidelity to the agreement (e.g., if he fails to give the health professional information she needs in order to give him optimum treatment), he makes it impossible for her to act effectively as his agent. Yet, she is unaware that she does not have this information. She is unaware that, to this extent, she is unable to act as the agent of her patient. Some part of her context is intelligible to her. She is able to act more or less effectively in this. But a great

deal of her context is not available—and intelligible—to her. This is particularly harmful because she is not aware of this lack of intelligibility in her context.

REFERENCES

Fowler, M. D. M., & Levine-Ariff, J. (1987). *Ethics at the bedside.* Philadelphia, PA: J. B. Lippincott.

Humphry, D., & Wickett, A. (1986). *The right to die: Understanding euthanasia.* New York: Harper and Row.

Husted, G. L., & Husted, J. H. (1995). The bioethical standards: The analysis of dilemmas through the analysis of persons. *Advanced Practice Nursing Quarterly, 1*(2), 69–76.

Husted, G. L., & Husted, J. H. (1997). Is cloning moral? *Nursing and Health Care, 18,* 168–169.

Kikuchi, J. F. (1996). Multicultural ethics in nursing education: A potential threat to responsible practice. *Journal of Professional Nursing, 12,* 159–165.

Nightingale, F. (1991). *As Miss Nightingale said . . . : Florence Nightingale through her sayings: A Victorian perspective* (M. Baly, Ed.). London: Scutari Press.

Orlowski, J. P., & Kanoti, G. A. (Eds.). (1986). Ethical moments in critical care medicine. *Critical Care Clinics, 2*(1), 1–6.

Orwell, G. (1945). *Animal farm.* London: Secker & Warburg.

Rice, V. H., Beck, C., & Stevenson, J. S. (1997). Ethical issues relative to autonomy and personal control in independent and cognitively impaired elders. *Nursing Outlook, 45,* 27–34.

Zoucha, R., & Husted, G. L. (2000). Is delivering culturally congruent psychosocial health-care ethical? *Issues in Mental Health Nursing, 21,* 325–340.

Preface to Chapter 6

THE CROCODILE PARADOX

One balmy day on a south sea island paradise, a woman was washing her laundry in the sea. Her baby was lying on the sand a few yards away. A crocodile lurked in the nearby bushes. All of a sudden, while the woman was distracted by a spot of bear fat on a lace scarf, the crocodile rushed over and snatched her baby.

The woman pleaded, "Please don't eat my baby." Crocodiles, as any crocodologist will tell you, are remarkably straight-forward, reliable, and sincere. To tell the truth, their attention tends to be narrow, and their awareness dominated by instinct and tradition. Nonetheless, they have a charming sense of humor.

The crocodile decided to amuse himself by offering the child's mother this mocking bargain: "If you can tell me what I am going to do, I will give your baby back to you. But if you cannot, I will eat your baby."

This was rather unkind because the crocodile was determined to eat the baby. If the woman said that the crocodile would not eat the baby, she would not be telling him what he was going to do, and so he would eat the baby. If she replied that he was going to eat the baby, this would be what he was going to do only if, in fact, he did eat the baby.

What a dreadful impasse! Hum. We will have to think about this—but not for long.

CHAPTER 6

The Power of Analysis Through Extremes

M any ethical blunders and harmful things are done in the health care setting as a result of a health care professional's choosing the wrong person with whom to interact. The patient **himself** is the wrong person when the actions he proposes to take are ethically unjustifiable.

Extremes analysis will establish, through the standards, the nature of the case. Awareness of this nature will be awareness of what is to be done, for whom it is to be done, and why it is to be done. Awareness of the right person for whom one ought to take an action is a precondition of awareness of what action ought to be taken and why. Analysis by the appropriate standards can then guide the awareness of how it is to be done.

The right beneficiary has been found if:

- His autonomy is such that a rational, controlled, and nonaggressive agreement can be formed;
- It is justifiable for the actions that are to be taken to be guided by his freedom;
- The demands of objective awareness are justifiably understood from his vantage point;
- His self-assertion rightly determines the expenditure of his time and effort, and ought to have input into decision making and choice;
- Benefit and harm are well defined by him and appropriate to the context; and
- His vision of fidelity (i.e., of the agreement) is appropriate.

The wrong beneficiary has been found when:

- His autonomy is such that a rational, limited, and nonaggressive agreement cannot be formed;
- The way he proposes to use his freedom in the context is such that it would not be possible to justify his decisions and actions;
- He cannot exercise objective awareness in guiding his actions;
- His irrational control of his time and effort would frustrate effective ethical decision making and choice;
- His understanding of benefit and harm is nonobjective and aggressive; and
- His vision of fidelity lacks respect for the rights of others.

ANALYSIS THROUGH EXTREMES

"When you have eliminated all that is impossible, whatever is left, however improbable, must be the case" (Doyle, 1930).

Extremes is a method of analysis through which a health care professional can clarify a bioethical context by identifying the relationships—the rights and responsibilities—of the people involved in that context. It involves carrying a situation to ridiculous extremes in order that issues become clear. While some dilemmas do not lend themselves to extremes analysis, it is a very powerful instrument for analyzing those that do.

Analysis through extremes is made possible by virtue of the fact that it is usually easier to determine what is the wrong thing to do than it is to determine what is the right thing to do. Determining the wrong thing to do greatly assists one in determining the right thing to do.

The discovery of that which is definitely wrong—that which is ethically "impossible"—is a powerful tool when what is definitely right is not self-evident and not easy to discover.

What is right and what is wrong is right or wrong in relation to the standards. To ascertain that a certain approach would be the wrong application of a standard helps one to discover the right application. Even where the right application of a standard is vague and unclear, the wrong application will probably be more evident. And its wrongness—its ethical impossibility—will clarify the right approach and the right application.

For an objective and contextual awareness, under ideal circumstances, the right thing or things would be visible, and the wrong thing or things would also be visible. This clear vision can be achieved by focusing in on the extremes of each standard taken as a right (e.g., the right to freedom, the right to objectivity, etc.). Through this, one can determine whether the ethical nature of the health care setting would be better expressed in giving absolute and complete support for each standard as a right to a certain beneficiary, or whether it is best that this beneficiary should enjoy no exercise of—no right to—the standard whatever. This will establish the nature of the case overall and the most appropriate actions to be taken.

The questions to be asked are: Which extreme—absolute support for a beneficiary or no support for a beneficiary whatever—will most perfectly:

- Maintain the rationality and objectivity of the agreement,
- Satisfy appropriate commitments and expectations, and
- Avoid the violation of a right.

Extremes analysis proceeds by determining what the final results would be of one person or another having absolute control over the exercise of each standard. This is in contrast to that person having no control whatever over the exercise of a standard. Through this analysis, it can be seen which alternative is more just and desirable. When this is determined, the ethical status of each beneficiary, and the actions that are, and are not, appropriate to the context will become evident.

CASE STUDY ANALYSIS THROUGH EXTREMES

In analyzing these cases, we will focus in on the context by determining for the proposed beneficiary (normally the patient), in the case of each standard, whether the beneficiary's complete control of the standard or the absolute control of that standard by another would be relatively more rational, more objectively desirable, and more justifiable. The following is an absurd dilemma in every way but one: It perfectly illustrates the nature of an agreement that a rational nurse would not make, and how such a dilemma ought to be resolved.

Case #1 Maggie, a nurse in the cardiac step-down unit of a distant hospital, enters the room of 23-year-old Peter, just as Peter's girlfriend is storming out. Peter's girlfriend is obviously angry. When Maggie approaches Peter's bedside, she sees that Peter's sutures have torn and he is hemorrhaging. Maggie explains the situation to Peter and tells him that she is going to take the steps necessary to stop his hemorrhaging. He tells her that he does not want her to stop his hemorrhaging. He has broken up with his sweetheart and he has nothing left to live for. He wants to die.

This puts Maggie in a dilemma. She has an agreement with Peter that she will act as his agent—to take those actions that he cannot. On the other hand, Peter has made a very unusual request of her. Should she take whatever steps are necessary to save Peter's life or, as the agent of her patient, should she simply accede to his wishes?

If we analyze this case, this is what reveals itself. In this case, should absolute consideration for Peter's **autonomy** be the guiding standard of interaction or should no consideration be given to Peter's autonomy?

Peter is a unique, rational animal. It is his rational animality out of which his uniqueness is formed. The course of action Peter proposes turns a whimsical, emotional state, which obviously he feels very intensely, against his rational animality. This course of action turns Peter against his own uniqueness. If his uniqueness is such that the emotions engendered by a romantic disappointment would inspire him to turn against his life, this is contrary to the essential nature of rational animality. Therefore, it is irrational. He ought not be supported in this, since no professional agreement could possibly demand irrationality on the part of a professional. No one, including the nurse herself, ought ever assume that her professional agreement should replace her human understanding with duties. A nurse must expect to encounter and accept unusual religious practices or personal outlooks to which people have dedicated themselves. But never a spontaneous whimsy like Peter's.

In this case, is it more appropriate that Peter should exercise absolute **freedom** or no freedom whatever?

The decision he has made would negate his freedom—an unhindered future—through his death. Since Peter has abandoned his freedom, it is appropriate that the health care professional give no consideration to his plans to destroy himself. This is the best possible and most logical course of action the health care professional can take.

Should Peter's perspective be regarded as absolutely **objective** and definitive and be given all consideration or as entirely nonobjective and be given no consideration?

When objectivity is reduced to the level of emotional stimulus and response, objectivity is abandoned. Peter, himself, has abandoned his objective awareness.

Should Peter's power to control his **self-assertion** be absolute, or should no consideration be given to Peter's power to control his time and effort?

Peter, himself, when he abandoned objectivity, abandoned his power to control his time and effort.

Should perfect consideration be given to the benefits Peter plans to pursue or should no consideration be given to this?

Peter sees his greatest benefit in abandoning all the benefits of his future life. In the context of his life, the harm he has suffered is nearly insignificant. He already has abandoned **beneficence** toward himself.

Should Peter's present state of **fidelity** to himself determine his nurse's action or have no influence whatever on her course of action?

Fidelity to an event—his suicide—has displaced fidelity to himself—the self that could live a long and satisfying life.

The bioethical standards are many things. Because of what they are, they cannot be out of context duties.

It may be that Peter's future life would be so marred by the loss of his sweetheart that his life would, objectively, be not worth living. But for the health care professionals attending him, it is impossible to see that this would be so. In Peter's present emotional state, it is impossible for **him** to see that this would be so. Therefore, while it might be a mistake to interfere with him, it is far more probable that the benefits the health care setting provides are better brought about by ignoring his wishes and restraining him—even forcibly if necessary—in order to get the hemorrhaging stopped.

Maggie has a responsibility to do for Peter what Peter would do for himself if he were able, but in his present emotional state he is unable to do anything **for** himself. She has a professional agreement with Peter. But no rational person would make an agreement with another to care for his life and health and, at the same time, let him die on what can only be understood as an emotional whim. Health care professionals are expected to be rational beings—the more rational the better. A person who is rational, whether health care professional or patient, cannot logically be expected to make an irrational agreement, or keep an agreement by taking an irrational action.

In most circumstances when a patient wishes to die, his wish is rational, condoned, and ought to be condoned. Peter's case does not fall into this category.

Resolution of the Crocodile Paradox

When the crocodile made his good natured but horrifying offer, this is what happened:

The mother replied, "When you offered me this agreement, the **implication** was that you would listen to my reply. You said, 'If you can tell me what I am going to do, I will give your baby back to you.'

"I cannot **tell** you anything unless you **listen** to what I say. You will not **hear** what I say unless you **listen** to what I say. So, what you are going to do is listen to what I say and then you will give me back my baby, because I told you what you are going to do." Immediately the crocodile lost his air of urbane gentility, and with a surly lack of grace, returned the woman's child. He had failed to consider the **implications** of what he said. That which is implied in a context is often the most important part of the context.

Nothing can establish the validity of a proper resolution nearly as well as drawing out the absurd implications of its contrary. The implication to be drawn from Peter's dilemma is quite obvious. Implications seldom are obvious, but quite often extremes analysis allows one to confidently draw out the relevant implication.

For instance, the implication of Maggie letting Peter die would be that bioethical interaction, in its most serious moments, can be determined by a hysterical, emotional tantrum.

Case #2   Elizabeth is from a large and well-to-do family. She is 24 years old and living on the streets. Her family has paid to have her admitted to many expensive, private, psychiatric facilities for treatment of her schizophrenia. Elizabeth always signs herself out. Since she is judged not to be dangerous, she cannot be held against her will.

Elizabeth's symptoms can be well controlled with psychotropic medication. However, she does not take the drugs and says she does not like the way she feels when she is on them. She writes beautiful poetry, and says she finds "my own reality" much more interesting than the boring and tedious life she experiences when on the medication. She prefers the friends she makes on the street to the dullness of "so-called normal people."

Her sister arranges to have her poetry published and sends the meager proceeds to Elizabeth. She is occasionally picked up for vagrancy, however, and brought in for treatment. Her parents are always contacted. Elizabeth does not maintain contact with them otherwise. Eloise, a social worker, has been assigned to her case. What should be done? (Davis, Aroskar, Liaschenko, & Drought, 1997)

In this case, should absolute consideration for Elizabeth's **autonomy** be the guiding standard of interaction or should no consideration be given to Elizabeth's autonomy?

Elizabeth is a rational animal, but her conventional reason has gone on vacation. She is living in "a world of her own." Nonetheless, the way she is living violates no one's rights. As far as we know, she is asking no one to make a commitment to her and she has no expectations of anyone.

A series of interdependent questions suggest themselves in this case:

How can the greatest potential harm be avoided and how can the greatest potential good be produced? Is it more desirable for Elizabeth to be happy in her world, than unhappy in ours? Should Elizabeth sacrifice her happiness for the sake of reason, or demand of reason that it serve her happiness?

Elizabeth can avoid the greatest potential harm—the loss of her happiness—by continuing her present lifestyle.

Happiness is, and unhappiness is not, desirable. If it is necessary, at present, in order for Elizabeth to be happy, to remain in her world, then this is her best decision, even, in a strange way, her most rational decision.

In this case, is it more appropriate that Elizabeth should exercise absolute **freedom** or no freedom whatever?

The ultimate goal of psychiatric care should be to bring Elizabeth to a state where she is able to control and preserve her existence and to flourish. (In this, the goal of psychiatry is no different than the goal of medical science.) At present, her activities do not threaten her survival. They allow her the only form of flourishing she can enjoy. In Elizabeth's strange and uncommon case, she has a right to absolute freedom.

Should Elizabeth's perspective be regarded as absolutely **objective** and definitive and be given all consideration or as entirely nonobjective and be given no consideration?

In this unusual case, there is an, at least apparent, conflict between objectivity and reason. In several cases cited in this book, the resolution suggests that the power to reason ought not be sacrificed for the sake of objective awareness.[1] This is particularly true when the revelation of a new objective fact would be so emotionally devastating that it would be impossible for the hearer to exercise reason. When awareness of an objective fact, in the immediate moment, makes it impossible to reason about one's course of action in the future, objectivity loses all value.

As an ethical tool, objectivity and reason do not refer to a person's ability to do crossword puzzles or balance a checkbook. Reason, and therefore objectivity, are tools to achieve flourishing and happiness. In Elizabeth's case, happiness would not be achieved by adopting a more conventional lifestyle. So, in a very relevant sense, it would be irrational for her to change her lifestyle.

If any way could be found to enable her to be happy in a different reality, then this might be acted upon. But, at present, there is no such way.

Should Elizabeth's power to control her time and effort be absolute or should no consideration be given to her power of **self-assertion**?

The arena of Elizabeth's life and her agency is maximized in her present lifestyle and the friends she makes on the street.

Elizabeth's life is more purposeful and much more interesting than the boring and tedious life that she experiences when on medication. It is a great temptation to try to control the lives of others or, somewhat more beneficently, to try too hard to help others control their own lives.

Sometimes the best thing to do is to do nothing.

Should perfect consideration be given to Elizabeth's plans to pursue her own sense of **beneficence**—or should no consideration be given to this?

Elizabeth's desire is to continue the lifestyle she is living now. And no way can be discovered that would enable her to experience her life in this way under different circumstances (e.g., living at home on medication).

Should Elizabeth's present state of **fidelity** to herself determine her course of action or have no influence on her course of action?

Elizabeth, in her own reality, is experiencing life in an emotional state that many people might envy. Considering the fact that Elizabeth's family is well-to-do, they might exercise fidelity to her by adding something onto the meager proceeds that Elizabeth's poetry brings to her.

Gentle coercion to induce Elizabeth to adopt a more self-controlled lifestyle, of course, is justified. Placing Elizabeth in a state of slavery to appearances is not.

The implication of compelling Elizabeth to conform would be that a humdrum and conventional lifestyle is an ethical standard. A standard so important that, in enforcing it, every individual standard can be violated.

Case #3   Jerry is an AIDS patient. He has a rare lymphoma with several large tumors in his abdomen. Jerry is responding to treatment and will probably be able to return to his home. He has asked his physician and his health care professional to keep his confidence. He does not want his wife or his homosexual partner to know that he has AIDS. The physician encourages him to tell his wife and lover, but Jerry refuses. He says that he is very careful about using a condom, and he does not want to upset his present lifestyle with his wife and lover.

Should absolute consideration or no consideration be given to Jerry's **unique** desires?

Jerry's disease has robbed him of many potential benefits he would have enjoyed without it. He is now imperiled at every turn. Whatever happens may strip him of one of the few benefits he has left. If Jerry were to lose the relationship he has with his wife and/or his lover, the quality of his life would be greatly diminished. In addition to everything he now faces, either loss would be a type of "little death." But suffering the little death of a destroyed relationship is insignificant in comparison to the real death that Jerry's wife and/or lover would suffer if he were to infect them.

Jerry's physician has no right to allow these two people to be placed in jeopardy based on Jerry's promise to practice safe sex. Jerry's nurse has an ethical obligation to speak out if this is necessary.

Should absolute consideration or no consideration be given to Jerry's **freedom**?

The uniqueness of a person's position does not give him the freedom to threaten another person's right to life. Even more so, it does not give a biomedical professional a right to cooperate with him in this by maintaining a life-threatening confidentiality.

Should absolute consideration or no consideration be given to Jerry's **outlook** on the situation?

One cannot develop as an ethical agent, and one cannot flourish as a human being, without taking certain actions and developing certain attitudes. One does not maintain an ethically developed attitude toward one's own life if one does not inform another person that his or her life is about to be placed in danger. By informing Jerry's wife and lover, the physician would honor his own life and, at the same time, fulfill his human obligation to them.

Should absolute consideration or no consideration be given to Jerry's **self-assertion**?

The range in which one has a right to exercise one's time and effort has rigid ethical boundaries. It stops far short of any action that would endanger the life of another person. The fact that one might be careful while exercising this action is not relevant.

Should absolute consideration or no consideration be given to Jerry's **benefit** seeking?

Jerry's physician has an opportunity to extend a significant degree of beneficence toward Jerry. This opportunity is very much outweighed by the harm Jerry's physician has the opportunity to do to the others.

Is absolute consideration or no consideration whatever due the health care professional agreement? What consideration ought to be given to the rights' agreement?

The biomedical professional/patient agreement is not an agreement to conspire together to violate the rights of others.

If Jerry can exercise absolute freedom, he need not ever take precautions. If he has no freedom, then, while he will be inconvenienced, no one's life will be placed in jeopardy. His view of the situation cannot be regarded as objective. Sexual passion is not noted for producing objective judgments. Only by breaking a confidence with Jerry can his wife and lover be endowed with an objective awareness to which they have a right. One's control of time, effort, and sexual passion seldom go well together. No one whose life is endangered can really be thought of as exercising self-assertion. Life must be given precedence over sexual passion. The benefit to Jerry is relatively trivial. The detriment to his wife and lover could be fatal. A health care professional has no right to exercise fidelity to a patient when this would violate the rights of a third party. Out of respect for his own life, the physician should exercise fidelity to potential victims.

The implication of maintaining Jerry's confidence is that a health care professional ought to keep his professional agreement, even if this means violating the rights' agreement. But if violating the rights' agreement is justifiable, then there is no ethical reason to keep the professional agreement. The rights' agreement is the foundation of the health care professional/patient agreement.

Case #4   Alfred came into the hospital 4 days ago for a coronary bypass. The surgery went well, and Alfred seems on the way to recovery. A few hours ago, his family was in to visit him. The room was filled with quiet conversation, and the family seemed to share a sense of intimacy.

It is now time for Alfred's first heparin injection. Lois, his nurse, has just come into his room to give him his shot. For no apparent reason, Alfred refuses the medication. Lois knows that Alfred's failure to take the medicine puts his life in jeopardy. She explains to him the reason for the drug and stresses its importance. On the one hand, Lois' reason tells her that Alfred should take the heparin. There is every reason why he should take it, and no apparent reason for him not to take it. On the other hand, Alfred is adamant. He absolutely refuses the shot of heparin. He also refuses to discuss the reasons why he will not let Lois give him the injection. There is no apparent reason why Alfred's freedom does not give him the right to make this decision. There seems to be an irresolvable conflict between Lois' reason and Alfred's freedom.

If you think about the ethical dilemmas that Alfred's case involves, three things are obvious:

1.   Justifiable ethical decisions depend, not on the facts of the ethical context, but on those facts that are known. Justifiable ethical decisions cannot depend on facts that are not known. No decision of any sort can be made on the basis of facts that are not known or on the basis of a person's refusal to recognize them.

2.   An ethical agent may often feel guilt over the results of a decision that was made on inadequate knowledge. The guilt the agent assumes may very well be worse than the unfortunate result of the decision. If the agent made the decision on an objective reading of all the knowledge that was available, the decision would be perfectly justifiable regardless of its results. Alfred ought to be fully informed concerning the foreseeable consequences of his decision.

3.   An ethical agent's reasoned beliefs are sufficient to justify ethical actions. There is nothing whatever that an ethical agent can act upon except his reasoned beliefs. There is no need for an ethical agent to do better than he can do.

The health care professional might invite Alfred to come along on an analysis through extremes. Lois might dialogue with Alfred as follows:

"You have every right to decide what is going to happen to you, but if you refuse the heparin, you may suffer a stroke or a heart attack. You may very well kill yourself or become paralyzed.

Do you want to make these decisions entirely alone without any expert input (**autonomy**)?

Do you want to make your decision without any knowledge of its consequences or what these consequences would mean to you (**freedom**)?

Do you want knowledgeable guidance? Do you want to look through the eyes of people who can see the consequences of different decisions? Do you want to control everything that goes on in this room or do you want to make it an informed cooperation? If you keep your thinking narrowed down to your present mood, you may change your mind when it is too late (**objectivity**).

If you give your attention to yourself and the circumstances here in this room, you will probably enjoy a long life (**self-assertion**).

Six-feet under, there is nothing to which you can react. You will never again react to family or friends. You will never decide on where you want to visit or where you want to go on vacation. You will never again drink a cool beer on a warm day or spend an evening reminiscing with your wife in a quiet restaurant (**beneficence**). (The best thing a health care professional can find out about a patient is those things in life he most enjoys. These are always useful as spurs.)

There are a lot of decisions you do not have to make right now. You do not have to decide where you want to go in the next several weeks or what you want to do. But I think you are going to want to be around to make those decisions.

Alfred, you will be dead a long time. How about taking a few years to complete a good life (**fidelity**)? Okay? (The offer of an agreement.) Let's get at it." (The assumption of an acceptance.)

If he still does not want to take his heparin, he may, in self-defense, reveal the reasons why not. Then you will have much more to work on with him. But hopefully, in this way, you can show him—without telling him—that the unique person he is, in the way he is reacting to his present condition, makes him the wrong person—making the wrong decision for himself.

To act otherwise would imply that force is a valid form of ethical interaction, or that his experience of comfort and control in the present moment is more important than his experience of comfort and control throughout the rest of his life.

DISCOVERY VERSUS CHOICE

The outlines of a context can be discovered by analysis through the standards. Analysis of potential benefits and harms—the most fulfilling exercise of the standards as virtues is revealed through their foreseeable consequences. That which will be discovered will be the lesser of two harms, or the lesser of two benefits, or the existence of a harm opposed to a benefit.

The ethically appropriate beneficiary can be discovered in the structure of the context by analysis through extremes. Not only this, but there is always the possibility that another dilemma, perhaps more important than the first, may be discovered through extremes analysis.

Extremes analysis will reveal what is certainly the wrong person, thing, time, way, extent, and reason.

When it is perfect, an agreement will be with the right person. When agreement is not with the right person, it is imperfect. That which would ordinarily be the right thing to do will be the wrong thing to do, and every category will be failed.

THE PERFECT BIOETHICAL AGREEMENT

One who is the right person when no right is violated becomes the wrong person when a right is violated. The right person, when interactions are in sync with the nature of the health care setting and the nurse's role, becomes the wrong person when interaction is out of sync. The right person under the terms of a rational agreement, when the agreement becomes irrational, becomes the wrong person. **Rights is a product of an implicit agreement among rational beings by virtue of their rationality not to obtain actions or the product of actions from others except through voluntary consent objectively gained.** When there is no possibility of an innocent person's rights being violated, when the agreement between a patient and the health care system is consistent with the role of the health care system, and when the agreement is free of irrational terms, the bioethical agreement is perfect.

The fact that extremes analysis has revealed one person to be the right beneficiary of ethical interaction does not imply that he is to be the exclusive beneficiary of ethical actions. Others must be considered, albeit, in an indirect way and to a lesser extent.

If one went from extremes analysis to an exclusive concern for the rights of one beneficiary, one would have discovered the context, only to abandon it. The purpose of extremes analysis is to establish the right beneficiary, and what is right for that beneficiary. It does not, and cannot, give one a license to ignore balance and proportion in relation to everyone else involved in the situation.

For instance, your patient wants to talk to you about the condition of his wife, but you see that the patient in the next bed, who is not your patient but is unattended, is in intense pain. You check and discover that he has not been given his pain medication. You arrange for him to get his pain medication. Then you go to your patient to discuss his distressful situation. A health care professional's agreement with a patient does not include the proviso that she will not assist someone who is in severe pain before consoling the patient with whom she has an agreement. This is an example of giving up a smaller good to gain a greater good.

You are about to give your patient his aspirin as ordered. He believes that this will help him to sleep. A visitor in the patient's room has a heart attack. You give the aspirin to the visitor. You would do this even if it meant that your patient would have to toss and turn all night. But then, after the person who had the heart attack has been treated, you would, of course, obtain aspirin for your patient. This is an example of giving up a smaller good to prevent a greater harm.

You go into a drugstore to buy medicine for your husband who will die without it. The pharmacist informs you that he will sell the drug to you, but only at a wildly inflated price—a price that you cannot pay. A dilemma arises: Under these circumstances, would you be justified in stealing the medicine from the druggist? Should the druggist or your husband be the beneficiary of your ethical action?

It would be understandable if you were to steal the medicine. Then, later on, you could reimburse the druggist the normal cost of the medicine. The druggist has an implicit agreement with his customers that he will charge a standard price for his medicine. He proposes to break this agreement. You hold him to it. This is an example of doing a smaller harm to prevent a greater harm.

You have promised your kids that you will take them to an amusement park. Your neighbor is rushed to the hospital. She must have a delicate operation and she wants you to go with her to help her understand what is happening during the process. Obviously, it would be more rational of you to make your neighbor the beneficiary of your action. But, because of this, you would certainly not conclude that you should never again take you children to an amusement park. This is an example of doing a smaller harm to attain a greater good.

GUIDELINES

Simple dilemmas do not always easily lend themselves to extremes analysis. They are simple because they consist in two obvious extremes. The best dilemmas to put through extremes analysis and draw implications from are dilemmas you are living through. Quite obviously, these are not simple dilemmas in relation to your present knowledge.

Freedom and objectivity for various reasons are the most powerful standards for extremes analysis. Most instances of analysis through freedom will reveal how freedom is to be exercised and if its exercise will produce irrational consequences or involve a violation of rights. Most instances of objectivity will reveal what justifiable decisions and choices will be achieved and whether they would presuppose an irrational agreement.

It is very rare that it happens when one analyzes through the extremes of two or three standards, that the others are going to show something different. After two or three, the others will follow suit.

Most instances of self-assertion will reveal what would motivate self-assertion—and whether this will result in excess or deficit—whether the agent's control of his time and effort is commensurate with the terms of the agreement.

Most instances of analysis through beneficence will reveal how the idea of beneficence squares with the nature of the health care system or whether it presupposes an irrational agreement—an agreement inappropriate to the health care system.

Most instances of analysis through fidelity will reveal what fidelity requires—whether, for instance, it might require a violation of rights.

The greatest value of autonomy is in confirming analysis through the other standards. There is a venerable philosophical axiom—*"Operatio sequiteur esse"*—that describes the fact that the characteristic actions of an existent arise from the nature of the existent. So it is with the nature—the autonomy—of a person. The knowledge of whom he is follows on and requires the awareness of what he does, and why.

Another effective way to discover the autonomy—the individual nature—of a person is through his passions.

The patient's emotional reaction to circumstances may be the most reliable indicator of the condition of his autonomy. Therefore, a flawed autonomy will be demonstrated by emotional reactions toward the wrong thing, or the wrong person, for the wrong reason, at the wrong time, in the wrong way, and to the wrong extent. This will reveal a lack of justifiable cause and effect actions and reactions (Aristotle in McKeon, 1941).

Autonomy is the interwoven character-structure that produce a person's actions, and that he experiences as himself. The fact that he is likeable and attractive or upsetting and unattractive is in the eyes of the beholder. It forms no part—nothing—of his autonomy.

Only an autonomy that produces irrational or coercive decisions and actions is a flawed autonomy.

NOTE

1. The alternative here is not a subjective awareness unrelated to objective reality, but objective awareness tied to a smaller context—a context with which a patient is psychologically and cognitively able to deal.

REFERENCES

Davis, A. J., Aroskar, M. A., Liaschenko, J., & Drought, T. S. (1997). *Ethical dilemmas & nursing practice* (4th ed.). Stamford, CT: Appleton & Lange.

Doyle, A. C. (1930). *The complete works of Sherlock Holmes*, Vol. I: *The sign of fours*. New York: Doubleday.

McKeon, R. (Ed.). (1941). *The basic works of Aristotle*. New York: Random House.

Beyond the Basics—An Extended Perspective

CHAPTER 7

The Bioethical Standards
as Lenses

T he ethical aspects of one's profession require that one acquire as complete an understanding of a patient's situation and as complete an understanding **of one's individual patient** as circumstances permit. In the health care setting, the analysis of the vast majority of ethical dilemmas one faces will require nothing more than gaining an understanding of the patient. In order to act as the agent of one's patient as a professional agrees to do, all one needs is the ability to understand one's patient.

When you can analyze and understand your patient, you will find the resolution of his dilemma right next door.

A DIFFERENT DOOR

Myself when young did eagerly frequent
Doctor and Saint, and heard great argument
About it and about, but evermore
Came out by the same door wherein I went.
(*Rubáiyat* of Omar Khayyam, 1983)

The experience that Omar describes is quite common for students of ethics. They never get across the room. They "[come] out by the same door wherein [they] went." They hear "great argument" concerning the nobility of duty or the glory of utility, and when the first joy of learning has past, they realize that they have learned nothing related to their lives or intentions. If they do not become aware of this, they are worse off.

Sometimes, there is an ethical dilemma of which you may be unaware. If you have ever been a patient, you can understand this because as a patient you know that the health professional is not aware of all the things with which you are dealing. But, as you gain an understanding of your patient, and you act from this understanding, you may very well resolve a dilemma without even being aware of the fact that a dilemma existed. This is much better than not being aware of it, not acting on it, and failing your professional responsibilities to your patient— failing to do for him what he would have done for himself.

In either case: Whether a dilemma arises, it is desirable that you understand as much as you can about every patient under your care.

We cannot know the psychology of another person directly.

Here again, the bioethical standards come in. They come in as lenses onto the psychology of your patient.

Using the bioethical standards as lenses enables you to see and understand other people. They enable you to see your patient as an individual person.

Understanding the nature of another person can be compared with understanding something like a piece of hard cherry candy. How does a child first come to understand the nature of a piece of cherry candy?

First, he sees an opaque redness. Then he can smell the cherry aroma of the piece of candy. He can feel its firm roundness; tap it on the table and hear its hardness. He can then taste its cherry sweetness. And now he knows the nature of a piece of cherry candy. You can understand a piece of cherry candy on a sensory level: You smell it, you taste it.

You cannot understand a person on a sensory level, not by looking at him or even by listening to him. But you can understand him, in the same way you can understand that piece of cherry candy. You can come to understand him by discovering the characteristics that make him what, or who, he is. The characteristics that make a person who he is cannot be grasped on a sensory level. But they can be grasped through the bioethical standards acting as lenses.

Your patient is a person and, to be understood, must be understood as a person.

All too often, a health professional looks on her patient globally as a homogeneous and undifferentiated living organism—more or less like herself. She understands herself inadequately and only with great difficulty. Therefore, in the short time she has, she finds it nearly impossible to understand her patient. But the person that is her patient can be understood as a living, thinking organism characterized by a high degree of autonomy—uniqueness. As a consequence, her patient, as an individual, will be structured by a definite potential for freedom, objectivity, self-assertion, benefit-seeking, and fidelity to himself. If you stare at your patient as an alien mass, you will not understand him. If you discover him as structured by the virtues characterized in the bioethical standards, and are open to these characteristics that make him who he is, you will find it remarkable how efficiently you can understand your patient.

The Chinese philosopher, Chu Hsi (1130–1200), one of the most illustrious thinkers of his time, advised that, "The effort to probe principle is naturally subsumed in the nurturing process—one probes the principle being nurtured. The effort to nurture is naturally subsumed in the process of probing principle—one nurtures the principle being probed. These two processes are inseparable."

Translating this into terms relevant to our purposes, Chu is saying:

As one engages in the nurturing process (especially health care), one must examine the principles that structure and motivate a patient (these are the standards of agreement and the elements of autonomy). This is an essential—defining—part of a nurturing process. In order to do this, one who would nurture must gain understanding of the principles involved.

The most effective way to come to understand these principles is to study them in those whom one is nurturing One nurtures these principles (autonomy, freedom, desire, etc.) in one's patient. This is the art of one's profession.

The Standard of Fidelity Acts as a Lens

If you would know your patient, look at the attitude he has toward himself. His attitude toward himself shapes who he is.

You ought to do what is best for your patient. This is difficult unless your patient wants to do what is best for himself. In order to know your patient, you must understand his attitude toward himself. You must know something about what he values, including how strongly he values himself—his fidelity to himself. If his fidelity to himself is weak, you may be able to strengthen it.

To do for himself everything he can do, he must be faithful to himself. To do for him everything you can do, you must be faithful to your agreement with him. If you are faithful to your agreement with him, you are being faithful to yourself, as a health care professional. At the same time, nothing you can do will better strengthen his feeling of self-worth and his desire to exercise fidelity than your obvious expectation of his fidelity to himself.

The Standard of Beneficence Acts as a Lens

If you would understand your patient, look at his nature as a benefit-seeking person—how he defines benefits and how he acts to gain benefits and to avoid harm.

His actions suggest his attitude toward potential benefits and potential harms. When you explicitly understand what his actions suggest, you will have the necessary ethical understanding you need to fill your ethical role successfully.

The Standard of Self-Assertion Acts as a Lens

If you would know your patient, you must look at how he reacts to the things that demand his time and effort and, if possible, why he reacts in this way.

He is a private individual, which means he owns **himself**. His time and effort—his life—is his own. His relationship to his life is intimate. His actions and motivations—his control of his time and effort—suggest who he is. Gain an understanding of his use of his time and his effort and you will know him quite well.

The Standard of Objectivity Acts as a Lens

If you would know your patient, look at how clearly he is aware of himself and how he engages with the reality of his situation. If you understand his reactions, you understand him as well as you need to understand him. It is important to know him in this way because he is dependent upon that reality for his life, health, and well-being.

A patient's behavior reveals much about his awareness of objective reality and, more important, his attitude toward it. You gain an objective understanding of him when you make this as explicit as the situation allows.

Objectivity is a value to everyone. It is especially a value to a nurse, even more than to a patient. But a nurse's objectivity is the best asset a patient has.

The Standard of Freedom Acts as a Lens

If you would know your patient, you must look at his freedom—what he can do and what he cannot do—and the purposes he has set for himself.

When you recognize how your patient focuses his attention, what he focuses it on, and why he takes long-term actions, this gives you—and your patient—a very great advantage.

The ways he uses his freedom—his evaluation of his present situation and the long-term actions he plans to take—reveal a great deal about him. If you become aware of this, you will have a far deeper understanding of him. You will interact with him better if you know who he is. And to know who he is—you have to understand what he does.

The Standard of Autonomy Acts as a Lens

If you would know another person—your patient, your neighbor or friend, your wife or husband, or your children, and if you would interact effectively with them, you must understand their uniqueness. You must know how this person is different—**how** he is **who** he is. You begin with the knowledge that he is an individual, reasoning organism. From this, you try to discover as much about him as you can—through the other bioethical standards.

Dilemma 7-1 During the performance of a laparotomy for the removal of an ovarian cancer, Dr. Richmond discovers the presence of precancerous gonads in Amelia, his 17-year-old patient. This is a condition (testicular feminization) that occurs once in every 50,000 females. Most women who have the condition are not gratified to discover it. Dr. Richmond believes he has a duty to reveal this detail of her condition to Amelia because "she has a right to know it" (Adapted from Minogue & Taraszyewski, 1988).

LENSES IN FOCUS

Ingrid, a nurse who works with Dora, makes an ethical analysis of each of her patients. She proceeds, consciously or implicitly, in this way:

She seeks to learn the autonomy of her patient. She does this by learning about her patient. She does not do this by examining her concept of autonomy. She knows that her ethical interactions will be with an autonomous patient. It will not be with the idea of autonomy that she carries around in her mind.

She seeks to learn the areas of her patient's desire for freedom. She does this, also, by learning about her patient. She does not reflect on the concept of freedom in her mind. She engages in ethical interaction with a person. She does not engage in ethical interaction with a concept.

She engages in a close analysis of the context. She does this in order to determine if, and where, she might harm her patient by stumbling over the standard of objectivity. She seeks to discover where her patient will benefit by receiving some item of information. Her patient is the center of her ethical attention.

She attempts to determine areas of her patient's life where he will desire control of his time and effort while he is in the health care setting. She begins with her patient. She does not begin with a narrow idea, such as the idea of self-assertion.

She stays on the alert for areas where she can do her patient some good. She stays alert for areas where she might do him some harm.

The reality is that, if we look at a problem, we become part of the problem; if we look at a solution, we become part of the solution; [and], if we look only at the problem, or only at the solution, we miss the vital link between them. The link, it seems, lies in human activity and relationships in every situation. (Tschudin, 1998, p. 53)

LENSES OUT OF FOCUS

Dora's center of attention, on the contrary, is on her vague understanding of the standards, and not her patient. She regards the standards as deontological rules. In ethical matters, she gives her attention to these rules rather than to the well-being of her patient.

Dora's process of ethical discovery is not governed by the nature of her patient's situation. She feels a responsibility to the standards themselves. The standards, as she understands them, and only these, possess ethical relevance for her. Used in this way, the bioethical standards make it impossible for her to stay in tune with the context.

Ingrid's use of the standards assumes that the efficiency of a nurse's ethical actions is measured by the benefit the nurse's actions yield. Since she assumes this, the center of her ethical concern cannot be abstract, ethical rules. The center of her context must be the nature and the needs of her patient. The center of Dora's context is a standard. Dora assumes that the benefit of a nurse's ethical actions is measured by the mechanical conformity of her mechanical actions to an externally related standard. The center of her ethical awareness is rigid, abstract, ethical rules. Ingrid does not attempt to benefit a standard. Dora does.

> **A nurse who works for a telephone-based service receives a call from a young man who reports that he is going to commit suicide and discloses his plan for the time, place, and method. The nurse determines the threat is serious and calls 911 in the caller's area. The emergency response team arrives in time to save the young man. After the caller recovers, he contacts the advice service, furious with the nurse for 'infringing' on his freedom to commit suicide. (Malloy, 1998)**

He shares Dora's ethical perspective.

The bioethical standards are **means to ends beyond themselves**. They are not ends in themselves. There is no way, in the standards themselves, to show that the standards have any value.

Fidelity is of no value to fidelity. Freedom cannot be benefitted by having its freedom respected. Obviously, these ideas are utterly senseless. But, they are ideas that, in one way or other, inspire many actions in the health care setting.

> **Bob is an elderly, feeble, senile man who has entered the hospital for diagnostic studies. On her shift, Dora cares for Bob, and Ingrid cares for him on hers.**
>
> **Bob wants to get up and ambulate. In the context of his condition, it is foreseeable that he might fall and injure himself. Ingrid quiets him, but does not allow him to ambulate. Dora, terrified by the term "paternalism," does allow Bob to ambulate. Bob falls and fractures his hip.**

Dora claims that the reason she allowed Bob to ambulate was out of respect for his right to freedom. In Bob's context, Dora's claim does not justify her action. She placed the well-being of "freedom" above the well-being of her patient. More often than not, the benefit to a patient in not being restrained outweighs the possible harm (Strumpf, Robinson, Wagner, & Evans, 1998). But this is context dependent. And no abstraction, including freedom, forms a context. Only the circumstances and knowledge of reasoning, desiring, and acting form a context.

Ingrid claims that the reason she did not allow Bob to ambulate was through a fear that he would fall and injure himself. Unless what she did took place in a very peculiar biomedical context, Ingrid's claim justifies her action. Ingrid placed the well-being of her patient above the well-being of "freedom."

It is often difficult to know where and how a standard ought to be applied. Rational, ethical action on the part of a nurse without reference to the nature of her patient—that is to say, without reference to the bioethical standards as lenses—is impossible. On the other hand, the bioethical standards, outside of the context, do not and cannot outline the context.

The context must determine the application of the bioethical standards. They are very broad abstractions, and some way must be found to bring them down into a patient's context.

Dilemma 7-2   Rodney is one of Julia's patients in the intensive care unit. He is dying from cirrhosis of the liver. Rodney asks Julia for a small drink of water. The order left by the physician placed Rodney on NPO because of the actively bleeding ulcers in his stomach and intestine.

Despite all of his medical problems, Rodney is alert and thirsty. He knows the probable consequences of a sip of water and yet continues to want it.

Rodney's physician is called in the hope that he will change the order. He will not. He says that he wants to be conservative and is afraid that the water would trigger more bleeding.

Despite this, Rodney still continues to plead for a drink of water.

What can Rodney's nurse do?

THE REMARKABLE NATURE OF THE BIOETHICAL STANDARDS

The teaching of the traditional ethical systems begins in childhood. These systems are designed for the purpose of external control and "socialization." They inhibit the free play of experimentation and discovery—activities that parents sometimes, understandably, find annoying. They replace the young ethical agent's need to understand the nature of his action with an automatic inhibitor of action.

The bioethical standards are not guidelines to action imposed from outside. They signify properties inherent in the nature of every human person. These properties are the innate and defining properties of a human life. As guidelines, they prevent "contradictions"—actions or interactions—that conflict with a person's power to act—his agency. The traditional systems are creations formed for the purpose of external control. The bioethical standards are not creations. They become objects of awareness through discovery. They signify internal and external realities that are essential to human fulfillment and flourishing.

Rules are, in the end, only rules. Mathematical schemes are, finally, only schemes. But the bioethical standards are:

1. A blueprint of the nature of human nature.

The uniqueness of a human individual is the uniqueness of her exercise of the standards as character-structures.

2. Descriptions of what it is to experience oneself as human.

To experience oneself as human is to experience oneself as being: A unique, purposeful, rational animal; able to initiate and sustain purposeful courses of action; necessarily engaged with, and dependent upon, an external reality; compelled to seek awareness and knowledge of the external reality; able to initiate within oneself independent thoughts, choices, and actions; having innate authority over one's time and effort; compelled to act in order to sustain one's life; capable of making and retaining decisions; and capable of maintaining and controlling a directed state of awareness within oneself and together with others.

3. Descriptions of what it is to experience another as human—what it is to be human in an interpersonal context.

The bioethical standards describe the psychological preconditions of thought, decision, discussion, agreement, action, and interaction.

4. Objects of awareness through which each person is able to communicate with, and understand, the internal states of others.

5. Assumptions of everyone who enters into an agreement.

Anyone who makes an agreement with another person is, at least implicitly, aware that the person with whom he makes the agreement is autonomous, free, and so on. This is why we make agreements with people, and why we do not make agreements with rocks, trees, or breezes.

6. Implied by the existence of individual rights because they are necessary and sufficient preconditions of individual rights.

7. The virtues (the meaning of the term virtue will be discussed in chapter 9) of an ethical agent—one's excellence as an agent; qualities of character that enable him to form and accomplish purposes; and moral assets of ethical agents.

8. Natural instruments that enable agents to sustain and enhance their lives.

9. Objective conditions of an agent's relation to every aspect of the external world.

10. "Critical indicators" of ethical thought and of everything of which ethical thought is a precondition (e.g., ethical decision/agreement/interaction/justification).

11. Avenues not only to the thinking of others, but also to introspection—to the psychological location where one meets oneself.

12. Basic reasons that rationally motivate ethical agreement and interaction.

13. Instances of (implicit) agreements that are necessarily included in every explicit agreement.

14. Standards of decision and action through which ethical decisions and actions are justified.

15. Preconditions of all thought and knowledge and the benefits humans pursue by thinking and acquiring knowledge.

16. Purposes that are gained through action.

17. Preconditions of the enjoyment of any value, including the value of life.

Life is a value that is enjoyed through the exercise of the standards. For instance, one enjoys the exercise of one's capacity for freedom. This enjoyment is the enjoyment of one's life. This exercise is the exercise of one's life.

18. "Sinews" connecting the living thing to his life.

The values that are obtained, the needs that are met through the exercise of the standards are, themselves, necessary preconditions for the survival of the standards in the living being, and the survival of the living being himself.

19. Objects of personal awareness that enable one to enter an ethical relationship—a relationship based on possession of these character-structures by oneself and the other.

20. Constraints on an agreement.

21. Instruments to evaluate one's ethical decision-making process.

22. Objectives of ethical action. Values that are gained through the exercise of ethical action.

23. The principles of human nature and development.

24. Principles of human action.

25. Indispensable ethical principles.

26. The necessary means to bioethical perfection.

That which is personally advantageous for a nurse is to nurture—as she was motivated to do when she made the agreement with herself that she would become a nurse. Odds are, when she made this agreement with herself—this decision—it was a decision to be an excellent nurse, and to nurse excellently—to act with virtue, and to pursue her profession virtuously.

If her agreement with herself was to be a nurse, and to nurse virtuously, then she ought to do this for her own sake and her own benefit. In this way, the motivations of her action will provide the maximum benefit for **herself** and for her patient.

Quite obviously, given the nature of the biomedical professions, every professional action is, fundamentally, an interaction.

Her excellence and success, therefore, depend, not only on herself, but also on her patient. The power of her interaction is, to some extent, dependent on the power of her patient's interaction. In order to maximize the efficiency of **her virtues**, she must be capable of strengthening **her patient's virtues**.

For her to interact effectively, her patient must be capable of and willing to interact. In order to **perfect** her professional virtues, her power to act well and successfully, she must be capable of increasing the strength of his ability and willingness to act well and successfully.

This she achieves through attention to the bioethical standards. It is a demand of her rational self-interest.

MUSINGS

We have established that:

- Nursing as an intelligible activity relies on the nurse/patient agreement.
- The bioethical standards reflect those aspects of human nature that make the nurse/patient agreement possible and desirable.
- The existence of the nurse/patient agreement implies the appropriateness of the bioethical standards as standards.

The standards serve as lenses to increase a nurse's understanding of her patient, and the effectiveness of her nursing and ethical interactions.

Every person is unique. So is every bullfrog and every waterfall unique. And every group of persons is unique.

The uniqueness described in the bioethical standard of autonomy is not the uniqueness of bullfrogs, waterfalls, or groups. It is the uniqueness of individual people.

The freedom described in the bioethical standard of freedom is the ability to pursue one's life and guide one's actions through objective awareness. This is a freedom only possessed by individual people.

Objectivity is a biological device whose purpose is the well-being of individuals.

Self-assertion, clearly, is the self-ownership of individuals. One defining characteristic of a group is the absence of self-ownership (Le Bon, 1960).

Beneficence is a value that benefits. Any value that benefits is a value that benefits individual persons.

Fidelity is a virtue that can be practiced only by individuals, one by one.

Wherever nursing has a logical foundation, it is an activity essentially involving individual nurses and their individual patients. Every other nursing activity (e.g., education, administration, research) is an outgrowth of this.

Eighty years before the birth of Socrates, an ethicist was born who was as great an ethicist as Socrates—or greater. He was born in China, and his mother named him Chung-ni, after a near-by mountain. He is that awe-inspiring figure known to posterity as Confucius (551 B.C. to 470 B.C.). He taught 2,500 years before the evolution of bioethics. Nonetheless, he had a message for nurses, and all those who would nurture.

He advised those who would nurture to, "Look closely into a man's aims; observe the means by which he pursues them and discover what brings him contentment; ask him to state his ambitions, freely and without reserve. Store away impressions. Study how to take advantage of his good points and overcome his weakness" (Confucius in Bahm, 1992).

His advice to nurses might be to:

Look into a patient's autonomy, which is revealed in his aims.
Observe a patient's objectivity, which is revealed in the means by which he pursues them.
Discover a patient's understanding of beneficence, which is revealed in what brings him contentment.
Examine his exercise of freedom, which is revealed in the quality of his actions in pursuit of his ambitions.
Note the quality of his self-assertion, which is revealed through the impressions of his behaviors.
Study his fidelity to himself, which is revealed in his good points and his weaknesses.

So many years ago, but Confucius' message was symphonological. Scant wonder, then, that nurturing, in its essential nature, is symphonological.

REFERENCES

Bahm, A. J. (1992). *The heart of Confucius*. Fremont, CA: Jain Publishing.
Chu Hsi, (1990). *Learning to be a sage*. (D. K. Gardner, Trans.). Berkeley, CA: University of California Press.
Khayyam, O. (1983). *Rubáiyat*. New York: St. Martin's Press. (Original work, 11th century)
Le Bon, G. (1960). *The crowd*. New York: Viking Press. (Original work published 1923)
Malloy, C. (1998). Managed care and ethical implications in telephone-based health services. *Advanced Practice Nursing Quarterly, 4*(2), 30–33.

Minogue, B. P., & Taraszyewski, R. (1988). The whole truth and nothing but the truth. *Hastings Center Report, 18*(5), 34–36.

Strumpf, N., Robinson, J., Wagner, J., & Evans, L. (1998). *Restraint-free care* (Series on Geriatric Nursing). New York: Springer.

Tschudin, V. (1998). Myths, magic and reality in nursing ethics: A personal perspective. *Nursing Ethics, 5*(1), 52–58.

CHAPTER 8

Apparent Conflicts Among the Bioethical Standards

A ctions that are ethically appropriate in relation to one patient at a certain time and in a certain way may not be appropriate in relation to another patient. Additionally, the same actions may not be appropriate to the same patient at a different time or if the actions are taken in a different way.

Nurses can and ought to use the bioethical standards as ethical instruments. However, two problems can arise for a nurse in her use of the standards:

1.   She can be uncertain as to the application of a bioethical standard. This uncertainty produces a dilemma.

2.   She can feel a greater confidence in the application of a standard than is justified. This feeling can block the resolution of a dilemma. It can leave a nurse with the realization that the decision she made was not the best decision, when it is too late. Equally unfortunate, she can make a bad decision without ever realizing it (Tuckett, 1999).

These problems arise because it is possible for conflicts to arise in the **nurse's understanding** of the appropriate application of the standards. We will now turn to those conflicts.

Dilemma 8-1   Fred is an 85-year-old man who suffers from senile dementia. He is depressed and aggressive. For some time, he has undergone antidepressant treatment, which has made it easier for him and his caregivers. However, he suddenly refuses to accept the treatment after he has heard that it is given to insane people. He says he is not insane and so he now refuses to accept the medication. There seems to be no way to convince him. His wife, who visits him each day, is desperate. She urges the physician who visits the nursing home to give her husband the antidepressant, by force if needed. She wants him to have the medication for his own sake and for hers. She doubts that her husband fully understands the consequences of his rejection of the medicine. The physician consults the nurse who is responsible for him, who agrees to use force. The antidepressant is given to the man by injection, while several people hold him down (Tannsjo, 1999, p. 329).

Here, then, is a conflict among several standards. Whatever resolution is possible, **it seems** it must come from outside of the standards. But then it would come from outside of the nurse/patient agreement—since that agreement can only be understood in terms of the bioethical standards.

But a nurse is the agent of her patient, doing for her patient what he would do for himself if he were able. This always takes place within a context. The nurse/patient agreement establishes the fact of this relationship. The **context** establishes the nature and purposes of the relationship and actions that can and ought to be taken. No other actions are ethically justifiable. And nothing can come from outside of this relationship. There are two possible approaches to a resolution. Both involve, in one way or another, the standards.

AUTONOMY AND FREEDOM

The standards of freedom and autonomy are often confused. They are not the same. A person's freedom is his ability to take independent actions. His *right to freedom* is his right to make independent and long-term choices and decisions and to act on these choices and decisions.

Dilemma 8-2   A health care professional is determined that a patient shall exercise his right to make decisions regarding his treatment. The patient wants the health care professional to make the decisions.

It can be argued that:

• The patient is exercising his freedom by delegating responsibility to the professional.

- The nature of this patient's autonomy is such that this is the best way he can exercise his freedom.
- A patient's relationship to a health care professional always, to some extent, involves this delegation of responsibility.

Also, it can be argued that:

- The patient is not exercising his right to freedom in refusing to exercise it.
- The patient is not expressing his autonomy, but abandoning it.
- In matters concerning the course of his life, it is ethically desirable that a patient delegate as little responsibility as possible.

In the life of a nurse, a large number of apparent conflicts arise between autonomy and freedom. They sometimes arise out of a failure to differentiate between the two.

The *standard of freedom* involves his right to take uncoerced actions, actions motivated by his own independent purposes and judgment. A biomedical professional's refusal to accept a patient's decisions and choices is a violation of the bioethical standard of freedom. The professional's efforts to coerce actions from her patient is another form of the same violation.

A person's autonomy is his independent uniqueness. His right to autonomy is his right to be what he is. Every form of intolerance is directed against someone's autonomy.

The difference between autonomy and freedom is shown by a consideration of the way each standard is violated.

AUTONOMY AND OBJECTIVITY

Patients sometimes experience a psychological disequilibrium, which interferes with their being able to participate readily in health-care decision making. They may retain the ability to think logically in other areas, but in this area, their thinking is distorted (Howe, 1993). Health care professionals need the ability to help these people see the consequences of ill-considered decisions. This is an ethical ability.

A nurse has an ethical obligation to recognize the fear of a patient who is more fearful than most. This is one way a professional recognizes the autonomy of her patient. Each patient has a right to be who he is, and some patients are more fearful than others.

Dilemma 8-3 Rachel is a nurse whose patient, Ken, is dying. She and Ken are old friends. Rachel knows that Ken is probably unaware of the seriousness of his condition, and she knows that Ken is terrified of dying. She also knows that Ken has many business and personal affairs that he would want to get in order if he knew of his condition. Rachel is, as the saying goes, caught on the horns of a dilemma. If she reveals his condition and incites terror in him, she will be ignoring Ken's present personality-structure. This would be a violation of his autonomy. If she does not tell him and enable him to get his affairs in order, she will be violating the standard of objectivity.

Since they are old friends, Ken might expect Rachel to tell him that he is dying. At the same time, his behavior might have given her no opportunity to do this.

But Rachel's behavior might lead him to believe that he is not dying, which is not true. If she knew that her behavior might mislead him and she could have prevented this, then, in respecting his autonomy, she violated the standard of objectivity. On the other hand, in respecting the need for objectivity, she may violate his autonomy.

Note that, whatever Rachel does, she must find some way to apply what she does know to what she does not know. Rachel is in a double bind. Neither autonomy nor objectivity will enable her to work her way out of this dilemma.

AUTONOMY AND SELF-ASSERTION

An individual person's right to self-assertion is an outgrowth of autonomy, an outgrowth of his "right"[1] to be who he is. One thing that every person is, regardless of other differences or similarities, is an independent individual. Every person is self-assertive by nature. One cannot deny (violate) the self-ownership of another without, at the same time, denying (violating) his autonomy. Nor, of course, can one violate the autonomy of another without violating his self-ownership. If a nurse rigorously accepts a patient's autonomy, she cannot violate his self-assertion.

Autonomy is individual and independent uniqueness. A person's right to autonomy is that moral property whereby he has the right to be dealt with according to his uniqueness. A person's right to self-assertion is his right to self-ownership— his right to control his time and effort, which includes his right to be free of undesired and undesirable interactions or relationships.

Dilemma 8-4   Ron works as a copyeditor. He is a 27-year-old homosexual with a long history of kidney disease. Three years ago, he tested positive for HIV, but he has been symptom-free and his T-cell count has been above 400. Ten months ago, he developed kidney failure, but since then he has been doing well on dialysis. He now wants to receive a kidney transplant from his 49-year-old mother, Mrs. Raymond. He has been very insistent that she donate a kidney for him, and she now agrees to the procedure. She knows that he is HIV positive. The psychiatrist who evaluated both Ron and his mother reports that they are both extremely guarded in their communication and that their relationship seems complex and troubled. The case comes to the Ethics Committee. Should the mother's consent be accepted as a free and autonomous choice? (Rhodes, 1992, pp. 75–76)

Like any conflict that arises between autonomy and self-assertion, it is not a real, but merely an apparent, conflict. The conflict arises only because one or both terms (autonomy and/or self-assertion) is ill-defined.

Mohan and his wife are asleep when their house catches on fire. Mohan manages to get out of the house. He is taken to the hospital in an ambulance. For a long time, Mohan cannot get information on what has happened to his wife. Finally, he is told that she is dead. He begins to cry. He asks Kathleen, his nurse, to see that he is left alone.

Mohan's physician is contacted by the coroner about arrangements for the disposition of the body of Mohan's wife. Mohan and his wife were Hindu and no one knows what should be done.

The physician instructs Kathleen to ask Mohan what he wants done. Kathleen tells the physician that Mohan is grieving and wants to be left alone for the time being. The physician angrily orders Kathleen to go and get the information he asked for. Now Kathleen faces an apparent conflict between an aspect of Mohan's autonomy (the fact that he is a Hindu) and his self-assertion (the fact that he wants to be left alone).

If Kathleen breaks in on Mohan's mourning, this will be a violation of his self-assertion. The only way it could be otherwise would be if Mohan does not enjoy self-ownership, but is owned by his physician, or perhaps, by his religion. That he is owned by his religion suggests that the autonomy that ought to be respected is not the uniqueness of Mohan, but only one aspect of his uniqueness— his religion. It suggests that Mohan can be dealt with, not according to his uniqueness, but according to the uniqueness of his religion.

The idea that Mohan's self-assertion might be the property of his physician is even more absurd. There is no way to make the idea that Mohan is owned by someone or something other than Mohan himself ethically intelligible. On the other hand, Kathleen would also violate Mohan's right to self-assertion. She would do this because his physician decided that the practices of Mohan's religion are more important to Mohan right now than his experience of the loss of his wife. This is not his decision to make. In asking to be left alone, Mohan made a decision from his autonomy concerning his self-assertion. If he has a right to autonomy and self-assertion, then, of necessity, he had a right to make that decision.

It might be argued that it is not Mohan, but his physician who decides what interactions Mohan finds desirable or undesirable. There is no reason whatever to believe that Mohan would order his priorities in this way or turn his self-ownership over to his physician in this context.

The conflict between Mohan's autonomy and his self-assertion is merely apparent. Both have been violated. There has been no conflict between them.

No even apparent conflict between autonomy and self-assertion is possible.

At least two other relevant series of events are possible here:

1.   Kathleen does not disturb Mohan. The coroner takes the body of Mohan's wife and handles it through the usual procedures. In this case, apparently, Mohan maintains his self-assertion, but his right, and his wife's right, to autonomy may be violated.

Surely there must be a conflict here.

But if we look at this series of events as it is, this is what we find. It is neither Kathleen nor the physician who violated Mohan's rights. If, in fact, anyone violated Mohan's rights, it was the coroner. Furthermore, note that no conflict between self-assertion and autonomy arises because the coroner does not become involved with Mohan's immediate control of his time and effort. Depending on other factors—the context of his knowledge, and the intentions that motivate his actions—the coroner may or may not be guilty of violating Mohan's autonomy (of course, he is not). But, even if Mohan's autonomy is violated, it is not Kathleen who violates it.

2.   It is possible that Mohan may require nursing and/or medical interventions. In this event, Kathleen must use careful contextual judgment. She must balance the importance of honoring Mohan's rights against the importance of the nursing or medical interventions.

If all Mohan needs to have is his morning care, it would be absurd for Kathleen to break in on his self-assertion. If he needs a vital medication, it would be absurd not to.

One does not have rights desire by desire, but in the context of one's life and over the whole span of one's life. One's rights are shaped by one's nature—and the context.

Whatever Kathleen does, she cannot escape a need for keen ethical judgment. No ethical agent can ever escape a need for ethical judgment.

AUTONOMY AND BENEFICENCE

Perhaps no ethical dilemmas that a nurse faces are more common than those that arise through apparent conflicts between the requirements of beneficence and the recognition of autonomy. For the biomedical professions as a whole, the most difficult and the most severe dilemmas arise through apparent conflicts between these two standards. These dilemmas do not arise in the context of the situation. They arise, whenever they do, in the context of the understanding, or more precisely, misunderstanding of the health care professional or her patient.

Dilemma 8-5   The classic case of a conflict between autonomy and beneficence is the case of a comatose Jehovah's Witness who needs a blood transfusion. His autonomy demands that, since he cannot explicitly communicate his wishes, it can be assumed that he would not want the transfusion. The standard of beneficence, on the other hand, demands that the professional act to bring about good. To allow a patient to die when he could have been saved is a very great failure to bring about good. Still and all, to give a patient a transfusion and save him, under these circumstances, might violate the standard of autonomy.

AUTONOMY AND FIDELITY

The primary responsibility for fulfilling the agreement between nurse and patient naturally lies with the nurse. It cannot be otherwise. The patient is a patient—one who is, to a greater or lesser extent, passive—unable to initiate action. Agency, the unhindered ability to initiate action, resides in the nurse.

Dilemma 8-6   Henry has a low tolerance to pain. He is very high-strung and fearful. He makes such demands on his nurse Irene's time and energy that she cannot adequately attend to her other patients. Does Irene's recognition of Henry's autonomous nature demand of her that she ignore her responsibility to her other patients? Or does fidelity to her agreement with her other patients override her obligation to recognize Henry's autonomy?

The ethical situation that Irene faces here is a dilemma that cannot be resolved by reference either to autonomy or to fidelity. The resolution demands a careful consideration of the definition of a nurse's profession (Husted & Husted, 1996).

FREEDOM AND OBJECTIVITY

An apparent conflict between the standards of freedom and objectivity can arise whenever two or more people are interacting.

Dilemma 8-7   Bobby is 4 years old. He has a problem with bed wetting. Bobby has asked Marilyn, his nurse, not to tell his parents, and she has agreed. Bobby's parents are, perhaps, overly concerned with his bed wetting. When his parents come to visit, they ask Marilyn whether Bobby has been wetting the bed. If Marilyn tells them the truth, this will be perfectly in line with the usual understanding of the demands of the standard of objectivity. It may also interfere with the spontaneous and positive interactions between Bobby and his parents. It will interfere with the actions Bobby wants to take. Instead of being open and accepting, Bobby's parents may be harsh and forbidding.

In order to facilitate Bobby's freedom of action, Marilyn would have to practice deception. She would have to lie to Bobby's parents.

One bioethical standard requires Marilyn to facilitate her patient's freedom of action. Another places a moral obligation upon her to deal with Bobby's parents on the basis of objectivity. The two together pose a dilemma for Marilyn.

The dilemma apparently cannot be solved by reference to either standard alone.

FREEDOM AND SELF-ASSERTION

1.   If any person enjoyed total and complete self-assertion, a question as to his right to take free action could not arise.

2.   But patients are in a situation where they cannot expect to enjoy complete self-assertion.

3.   If he had total and complete self-assertion, he would have no occasion to interact with another person. If he had no occasion to interact with another person, there would be no one to interfere with his freedom of action.

Responsibility with respect to a patient's right to self-assertion also involves a responsibility to respect his freedom. Self-assertion—a person's power and right to control his or her time and effort, and freedom—a person's right and power to choose and pursue long-term actions guided by objective awareness, are, obviously, intimately connected. But one does not necessarily depend upon the other.

Linda stops a former patient passing in the street to ask how he is. This is a way of interfering with her former patient's freedom of action, but it is an entirely blameless way. It is not a violation of his self-assertion.

This form of interfering with a person's freedom is of no ethical importance. Interruptions of a patient's freedom of action through an invasion of his self-assertion can occur in two ways:

1. Linda interrupts a patient's action even though the goal of this action is one upon which the patient places a high degree of importance.
2. Linda does not interfere with any important action her patient wishes to take. However, she subjects him to a constant series of minor interruptions. She violates his self-assertion simply by the repetition of minor obstructions to his freedom.

Occasions can arise when not interfering with a patient's action would mean a loss of his power of self-assertion. For instance, if a nurse would fail to interfere with a patient's actions when these actions will, foreseeably, injure a patient. There are also occasions when invading a patient's self-assertion will result in preserving his freedom of action. This occurs, for instance, every time a nurse wakes a patient (invades his self-assertion) in order to give him his medication (and thus enhance his future freedom to act).

A dilemma involving the standards of freedom and self-assertion could occur in this way:

Dilemma 8-8   A caller phones the nurse's station and speaks to Lotte, Ray's nurse. The caller tells Lotte that he is Ray's lawyer. He tells her that he was to come in today for Ray to sign his new will, but he is unable to get there today. He asks Lotte if he might come in the next day to see Ray. Lotte knows that there is a strong possibility that Ray might not live that long.

   If she tells the caller of Ray's condition, she may violate the standard of self-assertion. She has no way of being certain that the caller is Ray's lawyer. There is a definite possibility that the caller is a speculator who could use a prior knowledge of Ray's impending death to profit by undermining the value of Ray's corporation. If she does not tell the caller of Ray's impending death, there is a possibility that this will interfere with Ray's freedom to take actions that are vitally important to him.

   It will require a particularly keen attention to the context to resolve this dilemma.

FREEDOM AND BENEFICENCE

An apparent conflict between freedom and beneficence is a conflict in which a patient's desire to avoid acting stands in opposition to his well-being.

Dilemma 8-9   Margaret is 87 years old. She is very feeble, and is kept restrained in a wheelchair. She complains to Sandra, her nurse, that she wants to be "untied" so that she can walk around. Sandra knows that there is a very good chance that if Margaret were to walk around, she might fall. If she fell, she could severely, painfully, and permanently injure herself. This would cause her to lose the safe freedom of action she already enjoys. Untying Margaret would violate both beneficence and freedom.

Assume, however, that the only freedom Margaret could enjoy, since she cannot sit for any length of time, would be to walk around. A small change in the context changes a fairly clear-cut situation into an ethical dilemma. A minor change in the context will often have major ethical repercussions.

FREEDOM AND FIDELITY

Dilemma 8-10   Charlie, a heart attack patient, is having a heated argument with a business associate. He regards the favorable resolution of this argument as being of extreme importance to his career. Ingrid, Charlie's nurse, wants to call a halt to this argument, but Charlie wants to continue it. Ingrid believes, rightly, that this argument places Charlie's health and, possibly, even his life in jeopardy.

It is Charlie's life to do with as he wills. If Charlie has a right to live, then he has a right to take chances. Life requires one to take chances.

At the same time, Ingrid has had Charlie's health care placed in her hands. Her knowledge of the requirements of effective medical care is much greater than Charlie's. She has a responsibility to protect Charlie's life and health.

If Charlie exercises his right to take free action, Ingrid cannot exercise fidelity to her agreement. In order to exercise fidelity to the nurse/patient agreement, she must interfere with Charlie's freedom of action.

Nurses, generally, tend to argue in favor of Ingrid's right to interfere with Charlie. At the same time, they tend to argue against Sandra's right to interfere with Margaret.

But, in relation to the bioethical standards of freedom and fidelity, there are no fundamental differences between the two cases. From this perspective, these cases are identical. The difference is in the context. Each case places a patient's right to take certain actions in opposition to a nurse's responsibility to protect his well-being. Once again, the dilemma must be resolved by means of the contextual application of the standards. Nurses tend to argue rightly. Margaret is 87 years old. At this age, whatever pleasure and comfort she might gain is worth some risk, which can be minimized. Charlie is not 87 years old. If he is 47, he is risking, perhaps, 40 years. This risk cannot be minimized.

OBJECTIVITY AND SELF-ASSERTION

If a nurse is to defend her own right to self-assertion—her own right to self-ownership—she must take certain positive actions. She must actively maintain her right not to disclose any fact if this disclosure would threaten her right of self-ownership. If a nurse is to defend a patient's right to self-assertion, she must have the same attitude toward her patient. She must maintain her right not to disclose any fact when she is aware that this disclosure would threaten her patient's right of self-assertion.

> Two nurses, Sybil and Janet, work together and maintain a friendly relationship with one another. This relationship includes going out to dinner together occasionally.
> Sybil and Janet are both aware that, at some future time, together they may be in competition for the position of head nurse. This awareness has never before influenced their relationship. One evening, Sybil tells Janet that a mutual friend has said that Janet is a recovering alcoholic. She asks Janet if this is true.
> In fact, Janet is a recovering alcoholic. She can affirm that she is a recovering alcoholic or she can deny it. Or she can refuse to discuss the topic. If Janet does not deny this fact, or if she refuses to discuss the topic, then Sybil will have every reason to believe that the information she has received is accurate.
> It is quite possible that Sybil could use this information to prevent Janet's being considered for the position of head nurse. Then again, Sybil might never use the information in this way. It is very possible that Sybil is simply "making small talk" and is not at all thinking of violating Janet's right to self-ownership.

Janet faces a dilemma. If she tells the truth, and friends are justified in expecting the truth from each other, she surrenders her right to self-assertion. If she decides to maintain her self-assertion, she will have to lie to Sybil.

Let us look at a different situation:

Dilemma 8-11   Karen has entered the hospital and had an abortion. Her husband, Steve, a salesman, has been out of town. He locates Karen's nurse and asks her why Karen is in the hospital.

         This presents a dilemma. Karen's nurse knows nothing about the circumstances surrounding the relationship between Karen and Steve. If she tells Steve that Karen has had an abortion, she may be violating Karen's right to control her time and effort. If she does not tell him, she is violating the standard of objectivity—and probably for no reason. If she refuses to tell him anything, her refusal might cause Steve great anxiety. It might also sow the seeds of distrust in his mind.

It would be very desirable if a nurse had a way to deal with such dilemmas before they arose. But the nature of the context cannot be determined before the dilemma.

OBJECTIVITY AND BENEFICENCE

Apparent conflicts between objectivity and beneficence produce a great number of ethical dilemmas.

Dilemma 8-12   Hugh is dying. Lucy, his nurse, believes that his death is imminent. She remembers that Denise, his wife, had expressed a desire to be with her husband when he dies. Hugh and Denise had agreed to be with each other at the end so that the person who died first would not die alone. Lucy calls Denise to tell her of her husband's condition. It is a rather long time before Denise arrives at the hospital. Denise is blind and she must find someone willing to drive her to the hospital. By the time she arrives, Hugh has died.

    Before Lucy takes her into her husband's room, Denise expresses how glad she is to have arrived before his death. She spends several minutes in the room with her husband. She does not know that he was already dead when she arrived. If Lucy tells Denise that her husband died before she arrived, she honors the conventional standard of objectivity, but fails the test of beneficence. If Lucy tells her that she was with her husband while he was still alive, Lucy violates the standard of objectivity, but meets the test of beneficence. This poses a dilemma.

OBJECTIVITY AND FIDELITY

By the nature of things, conflicts between the standards of objectivity and fidelity cannot arise. Fidelity to the nurse/patient agreement entails objectivity in two ways:

1. The terms of the agreement must be objectively understood.
2. Actions that satisfy the standard of fidelity ought to be understood objectively.

But, in some unusual cases, a seeming conflict can arise:

Dilemma 8-13 Ike is Joan's patient. Ike's prognosis is poor. For reasons known only to himself, Ike does not want his wife Helen to be told of his prognosis. There are a number of legal and practical arrangements that must be made, and Helen needs to know the facts of Ike's condition.

If Joan reveals Ike's prognosis to Helen, she violates the agreement she has with Ike. Then she has lied to Ike.

But doesn't Joan have an ethical obligation to Helen? If she does not tell Helen the truth, it will mean an avoidable future hardship for Helen. Joan is not certain that Ike understands this.

Joan faces a dilemma that cannot be resolved either by reference to objectivity nor by reference to fidelity.

SELF-ASSERTION AND BENEFICENCE

Taken to the extreme, either self-assertion or beneficence would make the exercise of the other impossible.

If any person had the isolation of perfect self-assertion, it would not be possible for another person to act benevolently toward him, nor would it be necessary. If a person enjoyed perfect self-assertion—if he enjoyed perfect control over his time and effort—this would entail that he would succeed in achieving the object of all his actions. In this case, no one could act benevolently toward him. No one could bring any value into his life that he could not achieve in his own time and by his own effort.

Let us look at a more common dilemma:

Dilemma 8-14 Doris brings Shawn, her 5-year-old son, into a clinic to be treated for injuries sustained through a fall. Alice, the nurse who treats Shawn, recognizes that his injuries are much more consistent with battering than with a fall.

Beneficence seems to demand that Alice report her belief that Shawn is a battered child.

She cannot do this, however, without creating an invasion of Doris' self-assertion. Whatever she does, she ought to do it only with full awareness.

SELF-ASSERTION AND FIDELITY

A nurse has a moral obligation to remain faithful to her agreement with her patient. However, her obligation to exercise fidelity does not end with her obligation to her patient. As an ethical agent and as a nurse, she also has an obligation to exercise fidelity toward her colleagues and toward her employing institution.

Apparent conflicts between the standards of self-assertion and fidelity are rare, but here is one possibility:

Dilemma 8-15   Dan is in a nursing home suffering from Huntington's chorea. He will remain there until his death because he is no longer able to care for himself. He and his ex-wife have been divorced for the last 4 years. She comes in occasionally to visit him with their two children, Lauren (age 6) and Brian (age 9). Dan has made it quite clear to the physician and nurses that he does not want his ex-wife or children to be told his diagnosis. But if the children do not know of his condition, they will not be able to make an informed decision about having children of their own. Does Dan have a right to have his request honored?

BENEFICENCE AND FIDELITY

There are no conflicts between beneficence and fidelity.

A hypothetical conflict would take something like this form:

John is going to have his leg amputated. Suddenly, he changes his mind. He asks not to be anesthetized. Marilyn, his nurse, is determined that he shall receive the benefits for which he entered the hospital. The operation is performed.

Such an event, of course, could never occur. For this reason, no actual conflict between beneficence and fidelity has been shown.

For Marilyn to maintain fidelity to her agreement by coercing John into going through with the operation would involve an absolutely unjustifiable breach of his freedom. The agreement cannot be met in this manner. A dilemma that is resolved by coercion is not really **resolved**. A dilemma that is created by coercion is resolved by pointing out the coercion.

MUSINGS

The bioethical standards can ease a nurse into the bioethical context. They can make it easier for her to resolve ethical dilemmas. But conflicts in the **interpretation** of the bioethical standards can arise. When this occurs, they cannot be resolved in the context they have created. A wider context must be formed.

NOTE

1. Strictly speaking, every right is the right to take an action. To be what one is (e.g., a male, a redhead, a schizophrenic, or a hypertensive) is not an action. One does not act to be male, redheaded, schizophrenic, or hypertensive; this is simply what one is. The phrase "the right to one's autonomy" is not just a figure of speech. It denotes the ethical propriety of accepting the autonomy of any person with whom one interacts.

Not to accept the autonomy of another person is ethically improper since no one is ethically responsible for that which he did not act to bring about. No one ought to be praised or blamed because he is a male, redheaded, schizophrenic, or hypertensive.

REFERENCES

Howe, E. G. (1993). The vagaries of patients' and families' discussing advance directives. *Journal of Clinical Ethics, 4*, 3–7.

Husted, G. L., & Husted, J. H. (1996). Ethical dilemmas: Time and fidelity. *American Journal of Nursing, 96*(11), 23.

Rhodes, R. (1992). Cases from Mount Sinai School of Medicine, CUNY. *American Philosophical Association Newsletter on Philosophy and Medicine, 91*, 75–76.

Tannsjo, T. (1999). Informal coercion in the physical care of patients suffering from senile dementia or mental retardation. *Nursing Ethics, 6*, 327–336.

Tuckett, A. (1999). Nursing practice: Compassionate deception and the good Samaritan. *Nursing Ethics, 6*, 383–389.

CHAPTER 9

Virtue and Its Value

T he term "virtue," in its original sense, meant excellence. For instance, the virtues of a horse are its swiftness and endurance. The virtue of a physician is the ability to heal. The virtues of a wrestler are strength and skill. The virtue of a painter is the ability to portray.

In its classic sense, the virtue of a **person** came to mean all those excellences that arise from exercising control of one's actions through reason. This is the sense in which it will be used here.

Physicians directly serve and promote a patient's life, health, and well-being through medical interventions. This is the direct, immediate, and entire goal of a physician. The virtue of a physician is to do this excellently.

For other professionals, this is a mediate goal. In matters concerning a patient's medical well-being, a physician mediates between other professionals and the patient. A physician most often decides what is to be done to cure a patient. "It is the physician who cures and the nurse who cares" (Nightingale, 1969).

Ideally, a nurse would be one who has an immediate relationship with the person with whom she interacts. One small advance in the role that a nurse assigns to herself makes this possible. This advance makes it possible for a nurse to be more truly a professional, to provide greater benefits for her patient, and to derive the full benefits of her profession.

The nature of the health care setting and of nursing imply the nature of this advance. A nurse can make it her immediate goal to promote and serve the life, health, and well-being of her patient. She cannot do this by adopting the role of a physician. But she can do it by serving and promoting the **virtues** of her patient. This she does by nurturing and sustaining his power to act according to his nature—his ability to fulfill his **rational desires**. To a greater or lesser extent, many already do this.

The virtues of a patient are identical to the virtues of any professional or to the virtues of any other human being.

The virtue or excellence of a living thing is a form of well-being or power. It is the power, possessed by the living thing, to sustain its life as the kind of thing it is. Virtue, then, is a form of health (Aristotle in McKeon, 1941).

The ethicist, Benedict Spinoza, describes virtue thusly: "... reason demands ... that every person ... should desire everything that really leads man to a greater perfection, and absolutely that everyone should endeavor, as far as in him lies, to preserve his own being" (1949, p. 202). This is precisely what the health care setting is all about. Professionals can directly foster and nourish this aspect of a patient's health. A nurse, given the fact that she is with the patient over an extended period of time, can do this as no other biomedical professional can. She can be the custodian of his power to sustain his life as a human being. An effective nurse is a companion who interacts with, safeguards, and nurtures her patient's virtues.

In addition to everything else they are, the bioethical standards are the virtues of an ethical agent. They are characteristics of a person that enable him to sustain his existence as the person he is. They are qualities of character that enable a person to develop. They enable a person to act in order to fulfill his rational desires.

The bioethical standards, as virtues, are:

1. **Autonomy**   The ability to sustain one's unique and rational nature—those qualities of character that enable a person to be the person he desires to be. This ability makes one an excellent human being—one able to sustain his life as the person he is.
2. **Freedom**   The ability of a person to project and maintain purposeful courses of long-term action is an ability that makes him able to sustain his life and identity. This ability is a form of health and a virtue.
3. **Objectivity**   The virtue that enables one to perceive one's path to a greater perfection and to take the actions that are necessary for him to preserve his life. The ability to grasp and interact with the extramental facts of reality that are relevant to sustaining one's life and well-being is an ability that is a form of health and an invaluable virtue.
4. **Self-assertion**   The ability to dedicate one's time and effort to envisioning appropriate courses of action is a form of power that is a form of health. This ability is a profound virtue.
5. **Beneficence**   The ability to envision and take actions in pursuing one's benefit, or in acting to avoid harm is a power that makes one able to sustain one's life as the kind of being he is. This ability is a virtue.

6. **Fidelity** The ability to maintain one's self-awareness and one's determination to continue on courses of action that serve his life and well-being is a form of moral health, which is to say, it is a virtue.

A nurse ought to recognize these abilities as the virtues of her patient. She ought to recognize these virtues as her own. Imagine what a person's life would be without them.

Her justifiable interaction with her patient depends upon her motivating and nurturing his virtues. This is the meaning of " . . . acting for her patient as he would act for himself if he were able." Insofar as she acts as a nurse, her actions are justified.[1] They are also, as we shall see, invaluable to her as a person.

For a patient to sustain his life as the kind of being he is, two things are necessary. First, of course, he must sustain his life. It is the immediate responsibility of a physician to assist him in this. Second, he must sustain his awareness of the person he is. It is the natural and immediate responsibility of a nurse to assist him in this. The ideal health care setting will enable a patient to sustain his life as the person he is. This is the ethical ambience of medicine and of nursing. To achieve this ambience, both a physician and a nurse are necessary. Neither, alone, is sufficient.

THE BIOETHICAL AGREEMENT AND ITS STANDARDS

In one way or another, every ethical decision that a professional makes, every professionally justified action she takes in relation to her patient, involves the terms of the implicit (professional) agreement that establishes her dynamic relationship to her patient. Her practice is structured by it. A practice-based ethic—the ethic of this relationship—is derived from this agreement. It is based upon six noncontroversial but crucial points. These points are the bioethical standards. As we saw, they are presuppositions of the professional/patient agreement (and any agreement).

1. **The standard of autonomy** In order to grasp the terms of a specific health care professional/patient agreement, a professional needs to be aware of her patient's unique nature (autonomy). Every patient is a unique personality. To interact with a patient is to interact with a unique personality.

When a nurse acts as a researcher, an educator, or an administrator, she will not be aware of the unique characteristics of any individual patient. She must, however, always be aware of the unique characteristics of patients as patients. If any professional action, however indirect, is to be justifiable, it must be an action oriented toward the welfare of patients.

A great actress, to be able to perform effectively in a play every night, must rehearse her role. Only by rehearsing her role, can she perfect her performance. Every night, she performs the same actions with the same persons, and perfection requires rehearsal. The actress' role withers without rehearsal.

The situation of a health care professional is completely the opposite of this. Every day, she faces different moral demands; she must take different actions, with different persons, in very different circumstances. **A professional can only perfect her role if she does not rehearse it.** To perfect her role as a professional, she must meet the differing demands of every patient's situation. She cannot do this before she is in the situation. The delivery of ethical nurturing, in relation to each individual patient, is a role that cannot be rehearsed.

If an actress does not rehearse her role, she will never perform it other than "more or less" precisely. If a health care professional prejudges and rehearses her ethical actions, she will never make decisions and take actions toward a specific patient other than "more or less" appropriately. The life created by a playwright is entirely predictable. Life in the real world is unpredictable. The two professions require, for their perfection, two completely opposed approaches.

2.   **The standard of freedom**   In order to interact with a patient, a professional must interact with his freedom. Every action that a patient takes arises from his freedom. The precondition of a professional's interacting with the freedom of a patient is that she recognize and respect his freedom. A professional who fails to respect her patient's freedom is not interacting with her patient. She, therefore, fails to honor the agreement she has made with him.

3.   **The standard of objectivity**   In order for a person to interact within an agreement, he must understand the terms of the agreement. This understanding cannot exist unless the relationship between the parties is based on a rational trust, and rational trust cannot exist unless the relationship is based on objective understanding. Except in rare circumstances, a professional who does not communicate and interact with her patient on the basis of objective awareness violates the agreement she has made with him.

4.   **The standard of self-assertion**   All interaction presupposes a prior agreement between agents. An interaction that takes place through coercion of one party to the agreement is an impossible situation. If any person is coerced, there is no agreement and no interaction. A person can be coerced into doing almost anything. But no one can be coerced into making an agreement. No one can be coerced into interaction. No party to an interaction could possibly agree to be forced. If he agreed, he would not be forced. If he were forced, he did not agree.

Wherever there is agreement and interaction, there is the implicit presumption of the self-ownership and self-assertion of each person to the agreement. An agreement would be invalid if it, implicitly or explicitly, denied the self-ownership of one of the parties to the agreement. More than this, it would be a contradiction in terms. It would, in effect, leave one party to the agreement out of the agreement.

5.   **The standard of beneficence**   Every agreement has a purpose. This purpose is a goal to be achieved through interaction. An agreement without a final goal would be unintelligible. It would be an agreement to do nothing, and,

therefore, no agreement at all. The achievement of this final goal is the purpose of beneficent action—action that achieves a benefit. Every agreement, by its nature, calls for beneficent action. A professional who fails to act beneficently toward her patient fails to fulfill the agreement she has with him. This is a profoundly unfortunate failure. In this failure, a professional fails herself.

6. **The standard of fidelity** Wherever there is an agreement, there must be fidelity to the agreement. An agreement that will not be honored is a contradiction in terms. No professional can ever justify an ethical decision or action that violates the implicit agreement she has with her patient.

All these considerations form the ethical context of the interaction between professional and patient. The ethical effectiveness of this interaction depends upon the professional's acquisition of optimal awareness—the widest possible context of ethical knowledge—and on her bringing about, as nearly as possible, ideal conditions for what she and her patient intend.

All of this is facilitated by an increase in a professional's ethical awareness. "I urge you to be proactive in the best interest of your patients ... and stretch beyond your comfort zone" (Meyers, 2000, p. 9). It takes pride to stretch beyond one's comfort zone. Comfort and pride cannot live together. Pride is a most desirable virtue in a professional. Comfort (i.e., stagnation) is the only alternative to pride, and it is not a virtue.

THE SWAN PRINCIPLE

One fine day, two people, sitting on a park bench, fed the seagulls and swans swimming in a pond. One pointed out to the other the parallels between this scene and the health care setting, as the health care setting might be understood.

Some patients, like seagulls, are aggressive and demanding, while some are timid and lack self-assertion. While some are annoying, others are charming, some are resourceful, and others are helpless. It is easy for a professional's emotional responses to different types of patients to lead her away from the efficient practice of her profession. It is a temptation to avoid the demands of demanding patients, and to take advantage of the timidity of timid patients.

On a very basic level, seagulls and patients are very much alike. But patients are infinitely more complex than are seagulls.

Soon, the seagull feeders turned their attention to the calm dignity of the swans floating in the pond. They discussed between themselves how splendid it would be if nurses in their proper setting could achieve the self-assurance and serenity of the swans. The swans appeared perfectly placid and self-contented. They were aware of their circumstances and serene within them. Fanaticism of one sort or another, until it unravels, can produce an ethical assurance and certainty. But fanaticism is not a virtue. Only ethical competence can produce a reliable attitude of confidence and resilience. Without ethical awareness, professionals can be caught by surprise, and then their serenity and confidence are gone.

Ethical serenity and confidence can only arise from a professional's awareness of herself and her professional role. This awareness must produce a constant attitude, arising from, in Aristotle's words, a firm and stable character.

Living her role makes it imperative that her attitude be **focused on her patient**. As a professional, her role is that of "the agent of her patient doing for her patient what he would do for himself (through the exercise of his virtues) if he were able."

Every health care professional needs a framework to guide her professional practice. The clearer her state of professional consciousness, the more effective her competence. A framework will clarify her consciousness.

This framework is the ethical aspects of her role as a professional. The framework of her role, ideally, will be explicit—an ever present thought she can clearly express to herself. It ought to provide her with a constant, driving, motivating strength. Her explicit awareness of her role will take and keep her out of her comfort zone. It will bring her to a calm, swan-like, and reality-based dignity.

It will proceed somewhat as follows:

"My patient's virtues (autonomy) are such that he is moving (self-assertion) toward this goal (freedom) in these circumstances (objectivity) for this reason (beneficence). My virtues (autonomy) are such that I must act with him (interactive self-assertion) to assist him (his freedom) within the possibilities (of beneficence) in his circumstances to achieve every possible benefit that can be discovered (by objective awareness)."

Awareness of this framework for those professionals who are aware of it, unites and integrates their thoughts and actions—and makes their actions an extension of their thinking.

A topic to reflect upon:

Through her life, every professional is the agent of a patient, motivating and inspiring her patient to a state of agency, and guiding her patient's actions. **That patient, of course, is the professional herself.**

PROFESSIONALS, PATIENTS, AND CARING

Helen Keller, the famous lecturer and author, remarked that, "Life is a great adventure or it is nothing." Every professional comes into her profession expecting that it will be a great adventure. But sometimes, under the pressure of caregiver strain, professionals, especially nurses, become burned-out. When this happens, their profession stops being, for them, a great adventure, and becomes meaningless.

A professional who suffers from burn-out has lost her enthusiasm, her strength, and her endurance. She has stopped caring. Perhaps, from the beginning, her caring was flawed (Nelson, 1992).

"Caring is the essential fuel of a nurse's interaction with her patient. It is an essential means of understanding the needs and purposes of her patient. Without this, nothing can produce a successful chain of cause-and-effect interactions between them" (Husted & Husted, 1997, p. 17). Caring is the moral integrity of a nurse's [or any professional's] practice (Hartman, 1998).

Caring can open the way to understanding the needs of a patient. It cannot produce understanding of the ways to effectively meet these needs. Exclusive attention to caring assumes that there are only simple bioethical dilemmas, and that professionals can deal with these dilemmas instinctively. It further assumes that ethical dilemmas do not occur out in the external world of the patient, but only in the mind or the emotions of the professional. This is false. To experience caring is a virtue, to concentrate on caring is a flaw; in the same way, to concentrate on a standard rather than on a patient is an error and a flaw.

A caring perspective can replace an interactive relationship with a mere response. Caring, in and of itself, does not provide guidance. Guidance must be produced by an intellectual understanding of the patient in his circumstances. This understanding must be guided by logical consistency.

There is no reason why logical consistency cannot co-exist with compassionate caring. In fact, each perfects the other. Caring without logical consistency—caring for the wrong reason, in the wrong way, or to an illogical extent—will produce, as those who denigrate caring in favor of justice claim, injustice. Injustice to the patient, to the health care professional, or to both cannot be justified. On the other hand, logical consistency without caring will distort the whole reason for being of a health care system in a healthy society. This will, by that fact, produce injustice.

Caring can mean different, and even opposed, things, including:

1.   Sharing the values and motivations of another because they are values and motivations for this other. For instance, sharing a patient's struggles to regain his lost well-being through empathy for the patient.

2.   Being concerned with and attending to something or someone. For instance, sharing a patient's struggles to regain his lost well-being simply because he is one's patient.

3.   Undergoing mental suffering or grief. For instance, feeling overburdened from sharing a patient's struggle, and struggling with a patient as a burden.

4.   Being under the power of one emotion and devoting oneself to strengthening an opposed emotion. For instance, feeling overburdened from sharing a patient's struggle, and struggling to feel a concern that one does not feel for a patient.

Ways of Caring

There are also different ways of caring.

"Theatrical caring" is the way that one feels for a character in a movie or on a TV program. It is not a caring for a person. It is a type of play-acting. One rejoices at the success of a character-type—a patient. Or one is distressed at his failure. But it is not the patient as a person for whom one cares. It is a character in one's personal soap opera.

At best, theatrical caring is an exaggeration of common courtesy. At its worst, it is an unpleasant affectation.

Another way of caring might be called "reaction formation caring." This is when a professional tries to produce caring when she does not care—because she does not care. She is unwilling to admit to herself that she does not care, and so this kind of caring becomes a mask to cover her indifference. She cannot face the fact that she is indifferent to her patient, so she sees this mask as herself.

Reaction formation caring does little to nourish a patient and, for a professional, it is a process of self-deception and self-destruction.

A third way of caring is "codependent caring." This consists in a nurse trying to find her sense of ethical worth by working to make herself and her patient mutually codependent (Armstrong & Norris, 1992; Summers, 1992). It begins with self-sacrifice on the part of a professional. She escapes the need to think and understand by neglecting herself and focusing exclusive attention on her patient. When she finds her patient's response insufficient to fill her needs, she begins to feel victimized, resentful, and still dependent. Then, "compassion may disappear and a hardened facade may cover the nurse's . . . feelings of powerlessness, fear or shame . . . " (Summers, 1992, p. 70–71).

Through this way of caring, a health professional may attempt to find herself by abandoning herself. She attempts to fulfill herself by a course of action that destroys her (Morris & Trigoboff, 1992).

Another way of caring might be called "affinity caring." It is that which a professional feels when she shares the desires and purposes of the person for whom she cares. She cares for this person because he is a person and because he is this person. She cares for him because she values what he values and because she shares an adventure with him (Spinoza, 1949). This is the health care professions' great adventure.

Affinity caring is genuine caring. It nourishes a professional and her patient. It is caring for a person. This is the way of caring that health care professionals can be and ought to be all about.

Caregiver Strain

The problem of caregiver strain arises because of ethical dilemmas. What these dilemmas are is not important because caregiver strain itself is a dilemma. It is a dilemma that none of the traditional ethical theories will solve. In fact, it is a dilemma that any traditional ethical theory will exacerbate.

There is a process that can increase the emotional strength and staying power of a caregiver. If anything can solve the problems of caregiver strain and burn-out, this increase in strength and staying power can. For burn-out is the loss of emotional strength and staying power.

Under ideal circumstances, a professional will want to give care. A professional will want to see her patient's pain and suffering decreased through her efforts for a very personal reason. Pain and the loss of self-assertion are each forms of suffering (Spinoza, 1949). Ideally, a professional hates suffering in general, and specifically hates it as it affects each patient. A professional gains a deep sense of personal satisfaction simply by taking part in decreasing the pain and loss—the suffering—of another person, the person for whom she cares.

OBJECTIFIED ETHICAL ABSTRACTIONS

Caring, and a dedication to beneficence, does not require a professional to lose sight of herself or the facts of her life in order to share her patient's suffering. Ideal circumstances in the health care setting will increase a professional's self-awareness and strengthen her attachment to her life.

She can create ideal circumstances through the technique of orienting herself emotionally onto an objectified ethical abstraction.

"Objective" means existing in a context independent of the perception of a perceiving subject. For our purposes, "objectified" will be thought of as existing as a reality in itself apart from the concrete contexts in which it is found.

As we have seen, "ethics" means a system of actions taken in pursuit of vital and fundamental goals. Therefore, we use "ethical" to mean: Pertaining to vital and fundamental goals.

"Abstract" means mentally derived from individual instances. Tom, Dick, and Harry are individuals. By taking them together, the abstraction "men" can be formed. Tina, Doris, and Harriet are individuals. By taking them together, the abstraction "women" can be formed. By taking the (individual) abstractions "men" and "women" together, one forms the abstraction "persons." This action does not add anything to the external world. It simply adds to the mind's power of dealing with the external world. Therefore, by "abstraction" we will understand that which can only exist in and for the mind, but which can be thought of as if it existed outside of and apart from the mind.

Forming the Objectified Ethical Abstraction

In order to form the objectified ethical abstraction, a professional begins by observing her patient's suffering. Then, through an act of abstraction, she turns her awareness to many instances of suffering—perhaps her own suffering and the suffering of all her patients. She looks upon this abstraction, "suffering," as if it were a concrete thing in itself.

From here she broadens her abstraction to include all suffering—suffering as such.

Finally, she looks upon this abstraction—suffering as such—as if it were an independently existing thing.[2]

Now she has her objectified ethical abstraction—suffering.

Suffering is an abstraction because it is taken (abstracted) into the mind from every individual instance of suffering, and exists as an individual thing only in the mind.

Suffering is objectified because it is treated as a concrete thing existing apart from the mind. Suffering, as an abstraction, is an ethical abstraction. For the realm of values and disvalues is the realm of ethics. Suffering is that human disvalue the health care system was created to combat.

Interacting With the Objectified Ethical Abstraction

By interacting with the objectified abstraction, as well as with her patient, a professional's attitude is focused on more than the concrete present moment. The objectified abstraction gives the present moment a new and wider meaning. It enables a professional to relate to her patient without alienation on the one hand or codependence on the other.

By regarding this abstraction as concrete, her actions are motivated toward an almost visible entity. Her hatred of suffering and her consequent desire for the well-being of her patient are given a new strength and endurance.

It is impossible for any human to function without an awareness of abstractions. It is impossible to deal with Ethel's suffering, George's suffering, and Frank's suffering, as well as one's own suffering without being aware of the reality of that which is signified by the term suffering. If a professional is not spurred on by antagonism to the existence of suffering, her actions will be hindered and weakened by her unacknowledged awareness of suffering's vicious presence.

The entire purpose of the health care system is to help patients to overcome suffering, recover their well-being, or attain a peaceful death. Any professional who is not motivated by a hatred of suffering is out of sync with her profession—and her own nature. The absence of this motivation is not appropriate to a health care professional or a human being.

If one is enmeshed in the concrete, one cannot act effectively. One loses sight of the reasons for one's actions—the end result that is one's purpose. One's actions and one's purposes are made easier if one knows **why one is doing what one is doing**—if one has a firm idea of the end result being pursued. If a professional knows what she wishes to accomplish in general, and what she can accomplish here and now with this patient, the means to accomplish this become less tedious and stressful.

In one way, she is keeping her attention directed onto her patient, for she is combating her patient's suffering. In another way, by keeping her thoughts on the defeat of suffering and the victory of freedom from suffering, she is keeping her attention directed toward the abstraction of suffering.

This unites a professional and her patient by giving them a common enemy and a common goal. At the same time, it puts a psychological distance between them. This distance frees them from an unhealthy dependence on each other and does this in such a way as to bring them closer together.

This seems a strange, paradoxical result. But, before the professional formed her ethical abstraction—before she objectified suffering—she regarded suffering as a concrete object and took it instance by instance, up close. She was focused on her patient, who, in turn, was focused on his suffering. By focusing her attention on the abstraction, she places both the patient and his suffering back into perspective. Then she can see the health care setting in relation to her role and purposes, and her role and purposes in relation to this patient's situation.

Through this, **the professional and her patient are closer**. At the same time, she has a defense against caregiver strain. She has an emotional defense. She is not meeting this strain head on. She has distanced herself from the caregiver situation without distancing herself from her patient.

This distance, instead of hindering and sapping her action, gives her an abstract experience of the meaning and purpose of her action and gives her action long-term strength and endurance.

WHAT GOES AROUND ...

Most occupations or professions offer benefits peculiar to themselves. For instance, an architect can design his own home. Plumbers can avoid the (allegedly) exorbitant prices charged by plumbers. Surveyors are able to get out, into the outdoors. Accountants are able to stay in, out of the outdoors. Teachers have a wonderful opportunity to learn. Clowns are able to enjoy the enjoyment of children.

One occupation said to have a notable side benefit is that of the horse groom. There is an ancient saying to the effect that, "The outside of a horse is good for the inside of a man." This saying arose, supposedly, because horse grooms—those who care for the well-being of race horses—must give painstaking care to the horses in their charge. In addition to this, they have much time for themselves. Yet they are unable to travel far from the stables on any given day. This puts them in the habit of taking care of themselves. Notoriously, they tend to live a long life in good health.

There is also a notable benefit to be found in nursing. There is an approach to the profession that makes nursing the most rewarding of all occupations. **This approach offers a benefit that is greater than any benefit offered by any other occupation on earth.**

We have defined a nurse as, "The agent of a patient, doing for a patient what the patient would do for himself if he were able." A nurse must give counsel to her patient. She must also, as everyone must, give counsel to herself. As a nurse, she must inspire action in her patient. As a person—as an ethical agent—she must inspire action in herself. Throughout her entire life, a nurse is the nurse of a nurse. She is a nurse to herself. She gives counsel to and serves the virtue that is her own.

VIRTUES AND HAPPINESS

A health care professional ought to nurture and safeguard the virtues of her patient. Even more so, she should act to nurture and sustain her own virtues. If she does, she will enhance her patient's life. She will enhance the performance of her professional role. She will enhance her own life.

Ethics has to do with action and interaction.

People have a purpose in interacting: to maximize the power of their action. They interact because they can accomplish more through interaction than they can by acting alone. If people did not enhance their lives by interacting, they would not interact. They would have no reason to interact, as well as a strong reason not to interact.

People also act alone in order to enhance their lives. There is no such thing as a human action that does not make a difference. Every human action either benefits or harms the actor. Every action, properly so-called, is an action toward a goal.

Because of this, there is another reason why a nurse should nurture the virtues of her patient.

In recognizing and respecting the bioethical standards, a nurse safeguards the abilities of her patient's agency. To act freely, to make himself aware of the facts of his circumstances, to pursue benefits—these are abilities a patient shares with every human being. In safeguarding the abilities of her patient's agency, a professional honors her patient's rights. To be the person he is, to initiate action and to control his time, is every person's right. In honoring her patient's rights, a professional nurtures the virtues of her patient. In nurturing the virtues of her patient, she helps him to help her to succeed. She achieves virtue—professional competence—and excellence as a health care professional. These are one and the same.

In safeguarding and nurturing the virtues of her patient, in acting as the custodian of her patient's virtues, a professional creates and strengthens her own character.

First, she observes in her patient that a certain ability—a certain virtue—is needed. She does this by observing why that ability is needed. To observe that it is needed and why it is needed is the same observation. These are two perspectives on the same fact. These observations are the bridge between a professional and her patient. The ethical virtues are the bioethical standards—the standards of a professional's ethical action.

The experience of attending to her patient's virtues allows her to experience and to exercise her own. A professional looks into herself for her awareness of the virtues she must motivate and nurture in her patient. She will find these virtues in herself because, in filling her role as a professional, in working within the framework of her profession, she will have put them there.

MUSINGS

For a nurse, as a professional, far and away the most important agreement—the agreement that must precede any agreement she can have with her patient—is the agreement she has made with herself. A nurse who practices her profession without dedicating herself to it, practices her profession without dedicating herself to herself. (Husted & Husted, 1999, pp. 16–17)

This is the professional role a nurse, in particular, can make uniquely her own: To motivate, safeguard, and nurture the virtues of her patient. A professional can help a patient sustain his development and remain the unique being he is. She does this by maintaining her fidelity to her agreement with her patient and, through this, her fidelity to her patient.

In nurturing her patient's uniqueness, she sees the value of uniqueness and accepts herself as unique. In nurturing her patient's freedom, in practicing fidelity to her profession, she sees the value of freedom and teaches herself courage—the courage to accept and encourage her patient's freedom. In nurturing her patient's objectivity, she sees the value of objectivity and embraces it as her own standard. She achieves wisdom. She teaches herself to rely on all the knowledge she has gained through experience and to accept the fact that her knowledge is limited. This is the virtue of wisdom. In nurturing her patient's self-assertion, she sees the value of self-ownership and teaches herself integrity—a sense of unthreatened control over her time and effort. In approving her patient's striving for his benefit, she deals with him on the basis of beneficence. She sees the value of beneficence to him and to herself, and, prompted by reason, she teaches herself justice. In seeing the value to her patient of his fidelity to himself, she learns the value of fidelity and teaches herself pride in her profession and in herself. This is fidelity to herself.

She becomes aware of the value of the virtues to her patient. She sees his grim struggle to regain them. She learns the value of the virtues to herself. They are valuable to a person because of what it is to be a person. Virtue is the ability to be a human being. More than this, it is the ability to be a human being successfully.

By learning the value of the virtues, she learns the value of character. For a person's virtues are her character. From her patient's struggles, she learns the importance of destiny. From being a nurse she learns the matchless value of life.

When she comes to understand the value of life, she comes to understand the importance of destiny. When she comes to understand the importance of destiny, she comes to understand the value of character. By coming to understand the value of character, she gains an understanding of the virtues.

No occupations on earth can facilitate this understanding and the acquisition of these abilities more perfectly than the profession of nursing.

The French novelist, Balzac, warns us that an unfilled vocation draws the color from one's entire existence. Those who look for the glory of nursing in the right places will find it. Those who do not have looked for it in the wrong way.

NOTES

1. If the professional establishes a professional/patient agreement, she is, incidentally, most likely to avoid legal actions. Patients are not generally well versed on the law. Few patients ever say, "Looking back, I see where my professional violated the law. I am going to take her to court." Patients take health care professionals to court when they perceive a violation of her ethical responsibilities—when she has made them worse off than they should have been. If she is sympathetic to her patient's virtues, the possibilities of her being a defendant in a lawsuit are remote to the point of irrelevance.

2. Ordinarily, to do this would be to commit the fallacy of personification. This fallacy consists in attributing existence in external reality to an abstract idea. Examples of this would be: "History tells us that . . . " "History" tells us nothing—historians tell us things. "Medicine has come a long way . . . " There is no such being as medicine. "Medicine" is not a thing that moves from one time or place to another. The "long way" is a figure of speech meaning that medical professionals now have more skills and instruments than they had in the past. "Society demands." "Society" is not the kind of thing that demands. Only individual people demand various things.

Here, one is not guilty of the fallacy because one knows that suffering is not the kind of thing that one might bump into or meet face to face in reality. One only takes suffering to represent a concrete reality in order to generate the emotional attitude that enables a professional to avoid or overcome caregiver strain.

REFERENCES

Armstrong, J., & Norris, C. (1992). Co-dependence: A nursing issue. *Focus on Critical Care, 19*, 105–115.

Hartman, R. L. (1998). Revisiting the call to care: An ethical perspective. *Advanced Practice Nursing Quarterly, 4*(2), 14–18.

Husted, G. L., & Husted, J. H. (1997). Is a return to a caring perspective desirable? *Advanced Practice Nursing Quarterly, 3*(1), 14–17.

Husted, J. H., & Husted, G. L. (1999). Agreement: The origin of ethical action. *Critical Care Nursing, 22*(3), 12–18.

McKeon, R. (Ed.). (1941). *The basic works of Aristotle.* New York: Random House.

Meyers, T. A. (2000). Why couldn't I have seen him? *American Journal of Nursing, 100*(2), 9.

Morris, M., & Trigoboff, E. (1992). Co-dependence. In H. S. Wilson & C. R. Kneis (Eds.), *Psychiatric nursing* (4th ed.). Redwood, CA: Addison-Wesley.

Nelson, L. N. (1992). Against caring. *The Journal of Clinical Ethics, 3*(1), 8–15.

Nightingale, F. (1969). *Notes on nursing.* Toronto, Canada: Dover. (Original work published 1860)

Spinoza, B. (1949). *Ethics.* (J. Gutman, Ed.). New York: Hafner Publishing. (Original work published 1675)

Summers, C. L. (Summer, 1992). Co-dependence: A nursing dilemma. Revolution. *The Journal of Nurse Empowerment, 136*, 68–79.

SECTION 3

Advanced Issues

CHAPTER 10

Elements of Human Autonomy

It is inescapably necessary for every person to make and act on the basis of agreements. It is desirable for every person to understand the nature and the lives of the human persons who make agreements.

His desires—the things he reacts to, and how he reacts to them.
His reasoning—the ways in which he seeks, or fails to seek understanding.
His life—the way he sees himself in the present moment, his expectations of the future, and how he acts in relation to these expectations.
His purposes—the changes he is actually attempting to bring about in his life.
His agency—the successes and failures of his actions reveal this.

THE VALUE OF INTROSPECTION

These (desire, reason, life, purpose, and life) are the basic elements of individual autonomy. A reliable knowledge of a human person requires observation of that person. This observation, however, will tell us nearly nothing, unless we have first observed ourselves. We can only understand the inner world of another by beginning with what we find to be true of ourselves as human agents. We find this through introspection.

In order to gain understanding through introspection, a professional reflects upon herself, the meanings that things have for her, and how they came to have these meanings. To learn about another, she must begin with her own characteristics. Then, through observing others, she can discover what characteristics people have in common—the elements of human autonomy. After this, the only task is to discover how these characteristics are expressed in each individual person. This discovery will reveal the formative power of these characteristics in the person by whom they are expressed in action. This seems to present a dilemma:

Dilemma 10-1 Vladimir, a concert pianist, has sustained an injury that may affect his ability to play the piano. There are two operations that could be performed. One operation has a 90% chance of restoring gross movements of the hand and eliminating pain. Another experimental operation is showing about a 10% success rate in restoring fine motor coordination. However, if this operation were to fail, Vladimir would lose much of the gross movement of his hand. Vladimir must make a decision. The decision regards the possibility of achieving a value or the loss of a value. The value of being able to play the piano must be considered in the context of other activities that Vladimir values. The decision that Vladimir must make is an ethical decision. The action he will take, based on this decision, is an ethical action.

1. A knowledge of how the situation can guide the person's action in the pursuit of his purpose.

Vladimir must take into consideration these two essential facts: The success rate for one operation is 90%; for the other, it is about 10%.

2. A set of ethical principles held explicitly or implicitly.

When making his decision, Vladimir must consider the value he places on his ability to play the piano. He must also consider the disadvantages of losing gross motor coordination.

The situation can guide Vladimir's action through the ethical concepts that enable him to understand himself and his life. By means of these concepts, Vladimir can judge the relative desirability of both operations. We can assist him in this process.

In order to interact effectively with Vladimir, we will have to understand and get into Vladimir's ethical context—the context of his vital purposes.

THE DILEMMA OF THE HAMMER

A person needs an understanding of other people in order to understand him or herself.
But:
A person needs an understanding of herself in order to understand other people.

If both of these assumptions are true, then, it seems, no one can ever understand one's self or understand other people. One can never get started.

In order to resolve this dilemma, we will consider a much simpler, nonethical problem, one described and resolved by the ethicist, Benedict Spinoza (1949).

Spinoza proposes two facts, apparently contradictory to each other.

- In order to make a hammer, it is necessary for a person to be able to work iron.
- In order for a person to be able to work iron, he needs a hammer.

Therefore, it seems that no one can work iron, and there can be no such thing as a hammer.

For a person must have a hammer in order to make a hammer.

But a person must be able to make a hammer in order to have a hammer.

Therefore, it seems that it is impossible either to make or to have a hammer.

Yet, people do have hammers. People are able to work iron and to make hammers.

"Hammersmiths" began with whatever assets they had ready at hand, no doubt stones. They perfected these assets, more and more, until they had a primitive type of hammer. With this they were able to work iron—primitively.

The better they became at working iron, the better hammer they were able to produce. The better hammer they could produce, the better they became at working iron.

So it is also with ethical understanding.

Dilemma 10-2 Mr. Judd, age 64, comes into the hospital to have a tumor (later discovered to be benign) removed from his jaw. During the surgery, he suffers a cerebral vascular accident (CVA). Three weeks after the CVA, the physician asks the family about withdrawing food and fluids, and allowing Mr. Judd to die naturally. Mr. Judd has no living will or durable power of attorney for health care. His wife and children turn to Aaron, Mr. Judd's primary care nurse, for advice. On assessment, Aaron finds that Mr. Judd responds occasionally to simple commands, such as, "Squeeze my hands," "Turn your head," "Blink your eyes," and so on. Based on these observations, Aaron tries to talk to the physician. The physician insists that food and fluids be withdrawn. He believes that Mr. Judd will never get any better. Are there any further steps that Aaron ought to take?

A person looks into herself and gains a better understanding of others by observing how they are similar to, and different from, herself. Then she observes others and gains a better understanding of herself by noting similarities to, and differentiating herself from, others. (Or the process could be reversed—she may begin by observing others.)

This process continues and expands until the person reaches the fullest understanding she ever has of herself and of others.

A health professional begins by observing herself.

She observes:

- Her desire for autonomy—for the awareness of who she is and the power to sustain and develop herself.
- Her desire for freedom—for the power to act for herself in order to realize her own purposes.
- Her need for a true and objective understanding of her world.
- Her need to control her time and effort.
- Her desire to attain good and to avoid harm.

Through these observations, she gains a better understanding of herself. Then she observes others and discovers:

- Their desire to maintain their autonomy—the pleasure they take in being who and what they are.
- Their desire for freedom and the pleasure they take in acting on their freedom.
- The actions they are motivated to take to gain a true and objective understanding of their world.
- The pleasure they take in controlling their time and effort.
- The actions they take in order to attain good and to avoid evil.

Through this process, she gains a better understanding of her patient. She becomes able to act confidently and to justify her actions. The process continues and expands until she reaches her fullest ethical understanding—the widest understanding she is ever able to gain of herself and of her patient. The more knowledge she gains of herself, the greater the understanding of her patient. The more knowledge she gains of her patient, the greater her understanding of herself.

ANALYZING AUTONOMY

In our backyard, there lives a free-spirited bird named Ickarow. One day, some time ago, the way he tells it, Ickarow noticed that when he flies from tree to tree, the air presses against his body, slowing the rate of speed he could otherwise attain. Ickarow, oblivious to the need for analysis, has decided to fly up above the air so that he will be able to fly faster, more easily, and efficiently.

"Poor misguided Ickarow," we say. But is not a professional who hopes to arrive at an objectively justifiable ethical decision without a prior exercise of observation and analysis fully as misguided as Ickarow hoping to fly in a vacuum? She has lost her context as fully as Ickarow. She will never understand the ethics of her profession—no more than Ickarow will understand the mechanics of flying.

Ethical decision making must be preceded by ethical judgment. It cannot be any better than the judgment on which it is based. Before an ethical agent can know what to do, he or she must know who is involved and why it is being done. This knowledge is gained only through judgment. A perfected judgment is enriched by the elements of individual autonomy.

The autonomy of an individual is the unique nature of that individual. The elements of autonomy are the elements of human nature. They are the principles that make every individual person what he or she is. They are properties or characteristics possessed by a human person simply **because** he or she is a human person. They form the character of the person. They determine how a given person will experience and react to any given situation.

The elements of autonomy will serve the following tasks for a health care professional:

- They can facilitate her acquaintance with the character of her patient. If necessary, they will enable her to make a rigorous analysis of her patient's character and see into his values and motivations.

If a professional's objectives are to be met successfully, the road to success is understanding the patient's unique character. **The measure of her ethical competence is how well her actions reflect that understanding.**

- They enable a nurse to clarify the precise nature of the dilemma she faces.

The ethical aspects of the patient's situation profoundly involve from the way it affects him, the way he evaluates it, and in his reaction to it. Many of a nurse's ethical dilemmas arise when these evaluations and reactions are inappropriate to the situation. These evaluations and reactions arise from the way the elements of autonomy are lived by this patient.

- There are certain circumstances in which, for various reasons, the elements of autonomy serve better to resolve dilemmas than do the bioethical standards.

Generally, these will be when a nurse must do more than simply interact **with** a patient—when she must, in effect, also act **for** a patient.

The elements of autonomy are especially effective in the analysis of five types of dilemmas:

1.   When a nurse cannot speak to her patient, but must speak for her patient (e.g., when she speaks for an embryo or an infant; when her patient speaks a foreign language or comes from a significantly different culture; when her patient is comatose or otherwise incapable of communicating).

2.   When a nurse is acquainted with her patient's unique and individual nature well enough that she can actively engage the elements of his autonomy—his way of reasoning, his motivating desires, and so on, into her analysis. This is very rare.

3.   When a nurse joins a patient in deliberating about his future purposes and actions.

4.   When a marriage partner, significant other, or a parent wants to confer with a nurse regarding decisions for a patient.

5.   When her patient is a psychiatric patient. The elements of autonomy are the ethical bridge to a psychiatric patient.

No one can be human and be completely unfamiliar with that which makes him autonomous. Everyone is familiar with the elements of human autonomy, at least on an implicit level. It is quite advantageous for a nurse to become familiar with them explicitly.

DESIRE AND THE ETHICAL CONTEXT

Imagine a world in which desire is not a part of human nature. This world is a tropical island floating among the clouds. On this island, all the necessities of survival—fruit trees, cool water, and so on—are readily at hand. There is no motivation through discontent, no awareness that human life can be more than basic necessities. The faculty of human desire has withered away or the inhabitants of the world never possessed this faculty.

In this world, there are no specifically human realities. There are no human purposes, no human choices, and no human actions. In this world, every action is conducted on an animal level. Therefore, nothing is either good or evil. Nothing is either right or wrong.

In such a world, ethics, as a study, would be inconceivable. In this world where there is no human desire, there are no vital and fundamental goals. If there are no vital and fundamental goals, there is no need for a system of standards to motivate, determine, or justify these goals. Without human desire, human life would be unimportant. If desire were not an element of human nature, there would be no ethical realities of any sort.

Ethical realities exist in the world only because desire is an element of human nature.

DESIRE AS "THE ESSENCE OF MAN"

The great Dutch ethicist, Benedict Spinoza (1632–1677), said of desire that it is the essence of man. By "desire," Spinoza meant all of the physiological and psychological processes that constitute the life of an individual person. He defined desire as:

> [Desire is] that, which being given, [the person] itself is necessarily [given], and, being taken away, [the person] is necessarily taken [away]; or, in other words, that without which [the person] can neither be nor be conceived, and which in its turn cannot be nor be conceived without [the person]. (Spinoza, 1949, p. 79)

The term desire, insofar as it signifies an element of individual autonomy, has a specific meaning. It does not refer to any single desire for any single value. It does not even refer to the whole collection of a person's desires. It refers to, as Spinoza describes it, the defining fact of human existence. It is the nature or "essence" of every individual person (Husted, 1987).

This makes desire much more than simply a psychological reality. It makes every process of a person, as a living thing, an aspect of desire. From this perspective, **every** fact about an individual human being, and about all human beings, could, in principle, be explained in terms of desire.

Spinoza's definition perfectly defines desire in a professional context.

This point is so important, and so potentially valuable to a nurse in understanding her profession, that we will examine Spinoza's definition of desire on a simpler level than he presents it, and in detail:

- There is a minor difference in the chemical composition of males and females, but basically every person has the same chemical composition.
- Everyone's physiology is basically the same.
- Everyone has the same world to think about.
- Everyone's life depends on the same basic conditions.
- All people are limited, in the same ways, in the actions that they can take.
- Everyone has the same rights to life and action.

Despite all this, each and every person is different—is autonomous—in a vitally important way. There is one human attribute in which every individual person is different from every other. This attribute is human desire—as a psychological reality.

DESIRE AND THE NURSE'S ORIENTATION TO NURSING

A professional ethic, at all odds, should be appropriate to the profession whose members it is set to guide. Every profession arises out of human purposes and desires. Nursing, and the biomedical sciences generally, arose out of the desire to regain health and well-being, as well as to alleviate pain. Therefore, a nursing ethic ought to be appropriate to this desire. Without human desire regarded as **important**, what would be the need for nurses: What important human purpose could nurses and nursing serve?

A nursing ethic needs a logical basis for empathy with the desire to regain health and well-being. Without this basis, a nursing ethic becomes pointless. There will be no necessary and permanent connection between dilemmas and ethical analysis. Dilemmas will be subject to being resolved by convention and convenience.

An explicit empathy with human desire, as such, is the only logical basis for empathy with an individual's desire. If a nurse does not have empathy with human desire as such, she will not have empathy with a patient's desire for health and well-being. On what basis could a nursing ethic, for instance, approve of the desire for health and well-being, while not approving the desire for autonomy, freedom, and, ultimately, happiness? No health professional who lacks empathy with desire as a human reality has a stable empathy for any individual patient—or any individual person.

No bioethical standard is desired by a patient for its own sake. The reason for this is very simple. No bioethical standard exists in isolation from purposes to which agents direct it.

Chiang is in the hospital. His nurse, Evelyn, is quite aware of Chiang's uniqueness.

Evelyn's recognition of Chiang's uniqueness, however, is utterly valueless to Chiang. In itself, uniqueness is without any ethical importance. Uniqueness becomes autonomy—an ethical standard and concern—insofar as a person expresses this uniqueness by acting on his personal desires.

If Evelyn recognizes that Chiang is an accountant, a wood-carver, a husband, the father of two children, and that he lives beside a river, her recognition of Chiang and his circumstances is of no great ethical advantage. How could it be? The census taker who talks to Chiang in his workshop recognizes this much.

Another nurse, Jennifer, begins with the awareness that Chiang is motivated by desire. She recognizes that Chiang desires to earn a living, desires to perfect his skill at carving horses, desires to retain the love of his wife, desires the happiness of his children, and desires to return to his home beside the river. Jennifer empathizes with Chiang's desires. This fosters understanding between Jennifer and Chiang. It provides the basis for an ethical interaction between them.

A nurse will seldom, and perhaps never, encounter an ethical dilemma that she can resolve with a ballistic accuracy. Ethical dilemmas involving unique and "inconvenient" desires lend themselves, less than any other, to a clear-cut resolution.

Dilemma 10-3 Nine-year-old Wally was badly burned in a fire at his home. Iris, his nurse, comes to take him for debriding. Wally begins to cry and tells Iris he does not want to go. His face trembles, and he screams, "I'll go when my Mommy comes." Wally's mother was killed in the fire. Without any further discussion, Iris agrees not to take him.

The short-term benefit that Wally received by not undergoing the pain of debriding might not, all things being equal, compensate for the long-term detriment. But then, Iris must consider the possible effect on Wally if he is told, under these circumstances, that his mother is dead. Iris has, in a sense, done Wally some good. She may have done him greater harm. It is not possible to calculate the amount of good or harm that Iris has done Wally. The harm Iris did was permanent. Perhaps the good was also permanent.

Everyone desires to give and receive that which is good. Everyone desires to avoid that which is harmful. But in every concrete situation, it is not always easy to recognize what is good and what is harmful.

DESIRE AND ETHICAL DECISION MAKING

In a solitary context, what any person ought to do, among other things, is determined by what she wants to do and what she can do. What action she wants to take depends on why she is acting—the nature of her purposes. There are other principles of ethical action to be considered. But ethical decision making begins in desire—and is appropriately shaped by concern for every element of autonomy.

In an interpersonal context, there would never be any reason for ethical decision making if it were not for desire. Agents form an agreement and begin to interact. They need a way to define the purposes of their interaction. They need a way to keep their desires in harmony. The desire that originally motivated them provides that way.

SELF-PRESERVATION OF DESIRE

It is desire that brings a nurse into the nurse/patient agreement—her desire to be a nurse. The patient's desires are, so to speak, forced upon him. It is these desires that determine the decision a professional ought to make and the actions she ought to take. The desires that illness or injury force upon a patient make nursing what it is.

In one way or another, whatever a person does and whatever a person **is** are determined first by desire. The ethicist, Spinoza, tells us that, "Desire is the essence of man, that is to say, [desire is] the effort by which a man strives to persevere in his being" (1949, p. 201).

At one end of our existence, this desire motivates us to fill our basic needs. On the other end, it inspires the highest creations of the human mind.

But desire can be thought of as more than this. It can be thought of as the energy of life. All the processes that preserve and enhance the life of the organism arise from desire. From metabolism to reason, two forms of the energy of life, these processes serve to preserve and/or enhance the life of the organism. Reason does this fully as much as any other vital process. Reason, itself, can be thought of as a form of desire. It is a process that produces understanding. The achievement of understanding satisfies the desire for understanding. Understanding serves human agency and human life.

A person lost in a forest might feel a desire to create shelter for himself. He might examine all the resources about him and reason out a way to build a shelter. If he cuts his arm, the laceration will most likely heal itself. In several ways these processes—to feel, to examine, to build, and to heal—are very different. But they are alike in one very significant way. Each is a way nature has programmed the living organism to preserve its existence as a living organism. In a widened sense of "desire," each process can be thought of as a form of desire.

In the case of a patient, there is the most intimate connection between these different forms of desire. A patient's rational decision to enter the health care setting is motivated by his desire to regain his health. His desire to end the pain he suffers and to regain his health arises from, and is an extension of, unconscious bodily processes. These physiological processes are those that the body sets in motion in the healing process.

We can view the whole process—the healing processes by which the body regenerates itself, the conscious feeling of desire, and the reasoning process that produces the decision—as three expressions or steps of one natural drive. In one way or another, this whole process can be seen as the working of desire.

We can also view this process mechanistically. We can look at it as three different processes, one following on another and each moving in a different direction. If we do analyze the processes in this way, we view them like billiard balls striking one another on a billiard table. Then we have carved the patient up into three parts—a body, an emotional capacity, and a mind.

To do this would be in conflict with bioethical thinking. Biomedicine has begun to think of the patient as a unitary being—one who is to be understood holistically. It would also be in conflict with the patient's thinking. The patient is not a mind bringing a body into the health care setting. Nor is a patient a body bringing a mind into the health care setting.

If we look at humans holistically, we see their lives, as they live them, as conscious and embodied desire. In humans, reason is the instrument by which this desire preserves itself. Desire begins the process. Reason is the way that desire keeps it (keeps itself) going.

The biomedical arts are ways in which people preserve their lives. Medicine is the child of reason and desire.

REASON AND DESIRE

"Desire is, like fire, a useful servant but a fearful master" (Author unknown).

Every person is inspired by a desire to pursue the good as he sees it. The good is, as Thomas Aquinas observed, a form of the true. The true is the object of reason. The good is the object of desire.

That which can be good, however, is good only if it is true, only if it actually exists or can be brought into existence. The pursuit of the good ought to be guided by the knowledge that it does exist, either actually or potentially. It ought to be known that that which is pursued is truly good. This must be discovered by reason.

Ethical action is the pursuit of vital and fundamental goals. The goals of the health care professions are vital and fundamental values. For the health care professions, as for all ethical action, it is reason that makes the pursuit of these values possible.

Socrates said of reason that it is man's means to pursue the good.

Aristotle said of reason that it is man's means to happiness.

For the American logician and philosopher of science, Charles Sanders Peirce, reason is important because it is man's means of refining his beliefs.

For novelist-philosopher Ayn Rand, reason has ethical importance because it is man's means of survival.

Where there is good or the possibility of good in the world, where happiness is possible, where belief needs to be refined, and where survival is a problem that must be faced, there is an ethical universe. This universe calls for ethical action and practical reason.

In an ethical universe, desire is a human's source of action. Reasoning power allows a person to discover intelligible relations in his or her experience of the world. Reason allows the individual to adapt his or her actions in the pursuit of that which he or she experiences as good. In this sense, reason is the comrade-in-arms of all ethical action.

THE STANDARDS AS REASON AND DESIRE

A human is, in the classical definition, a rational animal. Imagine what your condition would be if you entirely lacked reason. Your relationship to your reason is so intimate that your condition, if you were deprived of reason, cannot be easily imagined. Without the use of your reason, you would have no more autonomy, freedom, or self-ownership than an earthworm.

It is through reason that nurses are able to consider the rationale for their actions, the scope and extent of their participation in decision making, and the manner in which decisions are to be made and carried out (Milstead, 1999). A nurse who totally lacked reason would not be able to understand or to act on the bioethical standards. She would, in fact, not be able to act on or to understand anything at all. To the extent that she does lack reason, or is unable to exercise it, she is unable to act or to understand. Even minor lapses of reason, such as occur under stress, may make it temporarily impossible for her to be guided by the bioethical standards (Rasmussen & Den Uyl, 1991).

Each of the bioethical standards is either a response to desire or is based upon some form of desire. In an ethical sense, each is also a form of reason or knowledge. Each standard **is** reasoning desire.

REASON AS THE BASIS OF THE BIOETHICAL STANDARDS

All a patient's choices, values, and actions begin in desire. A nurse ought to easily understand this. All **her** choices, values, and actions begin in desire. Those choices and actions that do not begin in her autonomous desire are not **hers**. Not surprisingly, she experiences them as alien. She experiences them as something outside of herself. The patient's experience of his desire is precisely the same. A patient, being in a state of enforced passivity, experiences most of his choices and actions as alien and not his own. He experiences them as being forced upon him.

A nurse has a significant advantage in understanding her patient if she understands this part of his experience.

Everyone's choices, values, and actions begin in desire. These, however, should not be allowed to continue in desire alone.

A professional's ethical thinking begins as a meditation on desire. But, very early on, it should be turned over to reason. This is true because of the nature of ethics—the structure of the world we live in, the nature of desire, and the necessity of reason. Ethical action is action toward vital and fundamental goals. Any action taken toward vital and fundamental goals must be sustained by reason. Otherwise, there would be no way for a nurse to know—and no way for a patient to know—that they are vital and fundamental goals.

Dilemma 10-4   Little Sandy is in the hospital to have his tonsils removed. Sandy is screaming and crying. He does not want to have the operation. The surgeon brings in the consent form for Sandy's mother to sign. Sometime later, Sandy's nurse gives him the preoperative medications.

This seems to be an easy case to deal with. It seems this way only because we take so much for granted. Sandy's tonsils are infected. It would be reasonable for them to be taken out. On the other hand, Sandy is already an autonomous individual. Autonomous individuals have rights.

At first glance, this situation seems to present no particular problems. Sandy must be operated on. All the same, ask yourself these questions:

1. Does Sandy's mother have a moral right to sign the consent form?
2. Does Sandy's nurse have a moral right to give him the preoperative medications?
3. Does the surgeon have a moral right to operate on Sandy?

Now, assuming that Sandy has no rights protecting him against this procedure (and, in every culture, we take it for granted that he has not), consider these questions:

4. When and how will Sandy acquire the rights that would protect him against this procedure?
5. Do Sandy's mother, the surgeon, and the nurse have rights that would protect them against undergoing this procedure involuntarily?
6. If so, when and how did Sandy's mother, the surgeon, and the nurse acquire these rights?
7. When and how will Sandy acquire the rights that his mother, the surgeon, and the nurse possess?
8. Will Sandy ever acquire the right to decide for his child? If so, when, why, and how?

We must assume that, at some time in his life, Sandy will acquire the right to decide for his child. If he does not, then neither did his mother ever acquire the right to decide for him. It seems as though reason is on the side of Sandy's tormenters. In reason, Sandy ought to have the operation. In reason, there is no reason for Sandy not to have the operation. There is no reason except Sandy's desire not to have it.

At the same time, it is a fact that Sandy is an autonomous ethical agent. If Sandy's autonomy will not protect him, nothing ever will.

The most rational course of action to be taken is for Sandy to have his tonsils removed. Can the reason why the others possess the rights they do be because reason is on their side? Does Sandy lack rights, in this circumstance, because reason is against him? Sandy's case shows the fragile interweaving of reason, autonomy, and individual rights.

It seems, then, that a conflict between reason and autonomy is built into the nature of rights. On the one hand, people possess rights "by virtue of their rationality." On the other hand, they can interact with others only if others give their "voluntary consent" to the interaction. This voluntary consent, in addition, must be "objectively gained." People possess rights by virtue of their capacity to reason. But they can interact with others only according to the autonomy of those others.

Conflicts can arise, even among benevolent people, over the question of rights. Most of these conflicts involve:

- One person's belief that reason demands or justifies an action.
- Another person's belief that this action would violate his autonomy—his right to be what and who he is.

Everyone has a right not to be aggressed against, coerced, or defrauded. This is the implicit agreement. It is the basis of ethical interaction. In addition to the universal rights agreement, a special implicit agreement is formed between nurse and patient. Special conflicts can arise here. Conflicts sometimes arise as to what constitutes aggression, coercion, or fraud. Although one person's reason tells him the other's rights have not been violated, the other's reason will tell him they have. Here autonomy must prevail.

Some middle ground must be found between the reasoning of one person and the autonomy of another.

Dilemma 10-5   Roger is an elderly man who was brought into the hospital because of dehydration as a result of the flu. While Roger is in the hospital, his physician realizes that Roger's pacemaker needs to be replaced. The physician and nurse go in to talk to Roger about the scheduling of the operation. After the physician leaves, Roger tells his nurse that he has no intention of having the operation. The last time he had a pacemaker put in, he suffered a stroke that left him confined to a wheelchair.

Even at his advanced age, Roger has autonomous purposes for his life. When he analyzes the benefit of having the pacemaker replaced (another year of life) against the drawbacks (the possibility of having another stroke and becoming completely dependent on others, or the possibility of not surviving the operation), he decides that his most reasonable course of action is not to have his pacemaker replaced.

On the other hand, when his pacemaker runs down, Roger may die immediately. This certainly seems to place reason on the side of Roger's physician. The physician feels, not without probable justification, that reason is on her side. The operation to replace the pacemaker would probably be a success and would give Roger another year of independent living. Whatever rights Roger has in this situation, he does not have them by virtue of any reasoning he has done. What Roger has to gain is objectively much greater than what he has to lose. It is almost beyond doubt that the course of action suggested by the physician is the course of action Roger should take. The physician believes that Roger is old and senile. She has Roger declared incompetent, and the operation is performed.

This situation places the rights that Roger has by virtue of his autonomy into conflict with the rights the physician has by virtue of her reasoning.

Ask yourself these questions:

1. Was the physician justified in the course of action she took?
2. Does a health care professional's role in society give her extraordinary rights?
3. What is the ethical role of a nurse in this situation?
4. The judge who declared Roger incompetent may have been legally justified. Was he ethically justified?

One final question:

5. Is there any significant difference between Roger's situation and Sandy's?

If reason is allowed to override autonomy in conflicts among rights, this will solve a large number of problems. At the same time, it will create an infinite number of problems. From then on, anytime anyone feels that his or her reason justifies a course of action, he or she will have a right to violate the autonomy of another. Under these circumstances, no one will have any rights at all.

If one is to have any rights, then reason cannot be allowed to override autonomy. Suppose that the reasoning behind one person's argument is superior to the reasoning behind another's. Ignoring the fact that, in most cases, it would be difficult or impossible to prove this, there would always be a third person whose reasoning is superior to the second. Then, there would be a fourth whose reasoning was superior to the third. This could go on forever. No ethical decision could ever be made.

Spinoza deals with the question of good and evil on its most basic level. He describes good and evil thus:

We call a thing good which contributes to the preservation of our being, and we call a thing evil if it is an obstacle to the preservation of our being, that is to say, a thing is called by us good or evil as it increases or diminishes, helps or restrains, our power of action. (1949, p. 196)

Reason and beneficence counsel a nurse to look at the issue of good and evil from her patient's point of view. Unless she does this, it is impossible for her to form and keep an agreement with her patient according to the purposes that brought him into the health care setting. This point of view and these purposes are the reasons why there is such a thing as the health care professions. A professional cannot ethically dispense with them in her ethical decision making.

LIFE AS THE PRECONDITION OF ALL ACTION

We have already defined desire to include much more than the well-known psychological state. A nurse understands her patient best if, by desire, she understands all the processes that contribute to her patient's survival and the enhancement of his life. The psychological state of desire is the best-known process of this type, but every process that contributes to the survival of the organism belongs to the same family.

By including every such process under the concept of desire, a nurse can have a well-balanced understanding of her patient. The patient's psychological state is only a small part of the context. Only this understanding of his desire enables the professional to interact with her patient in his entire context. This understanding of desire, as an element of autonomy, is an understanding of a person. For a nurse to know her patient as a living reality is at least as important as it is for her to know any isolated psychological state.

THE DIFFERENT ASPECTS OF LIFE

To gain understanding of the role of life in ethics, we must define "life" inclusively, in the same way we define desire. As an ethical element, life includes the entire context of a living person. As we shall see, any narrower definition would not be adequate for an effective bioethics. Under life, we must understand every process and action, including reason and desire, by which an organism maintains its survival and enhances its state of being.

We have a very limited understanding of life if we look at it only as a natural curiosity. We have an adequate understanding of life only if we understand it from the perspective of the subject who is living it. In order to do this, it is desirable to understand life from our own perspective.

For bioethics, an adequate understanding of life will include such things as:

- The body's physiological processes;
- The integration of these processes;
- Basic needs common to all animals—food, water, air—the needs that are directly and immediately tied to the animal's survival;
- Basic needs common to all human beings: Shelter, clothing, companionship, freedom from pain, etc.;
- The life of consciousness: Perceptual experience, conceptual thought, emotion, etc.;
- The higher-order needs and values of human beings: Purpose, creativity, hope, self-ownership, etc.—the values that are directly and immediately tied to a human level of existence;
- The value of various activities: Walking, flying an airplane, cooking, working, etc.—conditions of physical self-expression;
- The meaning of "aesthetic" values: Music, reading, painting, hobbies, discussion, etc.—those conditions under which a person examines and/or experiences his life at its best; and
- That with which a person is engaged and to which he is committed—the meaning, to a person, of the products of his acts of choice.

A nurse can define life from the perspective of an outsider. There are, however, a number of reasons why she ought to define life from the perspective of the living subject.

1.   Medical science defines it from this perspective. If medical science thought of life simply as physiological survival, there would be no such thing as psychiatry, physical therapy, plastic surgery, etc.

2.   If a nurse defines her patient's life solely in terms of its basic physiological processes, she will never be able to deal with ethical questions concerning risk, euthanasia, abortion, cloning, and so forth. If she defines life in terms of its basic physiological processes, then she will never truly experience her patient. She will be very much in the position of a novelist who, when she looks out at the characters in her novel, never really sees beyond herself.

3.   If life, as an ethical concept, were defined in terms of physiological processes, then life as an ethical concept would pertain to all organic matter.

All organic matter is characterized by physiological processes. All organic matter has basic needs that must be met if it is to survive. If a nurse narrowed her understanding of life as an ethical concept, to denote only physiological processes, she would have to broaden her understanding to include all living matter in her ethical concern. If she concerned herself with the freedom, self-assertion, and so on of all organic matter, she, herself, could not survive. Nurses, in common with everyone else, need to consume organic matter in order to remain alive. It would be strange indeed if a bioethical standard logically demanded the self-destruction of the health care professional who recognized it.

A nurse's ethical concern is not with organic matter, it is with a patient. It must be with a patient in his entirety. This is the only kind of patients there are, patients in their entirety.

Her ethical commitment to her patient does not arise from the fact that he is organic matter. It arises from, and is formed by, the fact that his life is all the things it is. A patient's life is his autonomy. In addition to his physical needs and processes, his life is his desire, his reason, his purposes, and his power of agency.

4.   If, on the other hand, a nurse defines her patient's life entirely in *abstract* terms, she will never be able to deal with her patient on an ethical level. People involved in ethical interaction are individual and concrete. Only an understanding of life as one element of an individual patient's autonomy will serve to guide ethical action. People are too different and life is too many things for the individual to be understood in entirely abstract terms.

It is not possible for a nurse to deal with her patient's life entirely on an abstract level. If it were possible, then she would hardly have to deal with her patient at all.

Only if a nurse defines the life of her patient as she defines her own life will she look at her patient as an ethical agent looks at another person in an effective ethical interaction.

A nurse's agreement is not with organic matter. Nor is the life that is at the center of her agreement a disconnected abstraction. Her agreement is with every aspect of an individual human being.

LIFE AS THE BASIS OF THE BIOETHICAL STANDARDS

A health care ethic that is not appropriate to patients—and to health professionals—is riddled with problems. The chief problem is that it is not an intelligible field of study. Not every ethical system is automatically intelligible. Ethics is, or ought to be, derived from a study of individual people as living, rational beings. There is no intelligible ethic of redheads or of diabetics. There is no intelligible ethic of poets or of long-distance runners. An intelligible ethic relevant only to males or only to females is an impossibility. Such an ethic would be a mistake or a prejudice masquerading as an ethical system.

A rational, solitary ethic is one whose motivations can be justified by the benefit it brings to the person who follows it. A rational, interpersonal ethic is one whose motivations can be justified by reference to the benefits and harmony it brings to the interaction of the people who are guided by it.

Human survival, on every level, is contingent upon rational belief. Rules and conventions are not substitutes for rational belief. They weaken the conditions of human survival.

LIFE AS THE PRECONDITION OF ALL VALUES

Nothing can be sought or desired by anyone unless that person is alive. Life is the precondition of all values. As ethicist Benedict Spinoza (1949) describes it:

> No one can desire to be happy, to act well, and to live well, who does not at the same time desire to be, to act, and to live, that is to say, actually to exist (p. 204).

In the field of ethics, one faces two options:

- One can choose a ritualistic ethic. This is an ethic based upon and arising out of rules and conventions.
- One can choose a symphonological ethic. For a health care professional, a symphonological ethic is an ethic based on her patient's purposes as codified in the nurse/patient agreement.

Nursing is far more intelligible under a symphonological ethic.

If a nurse follows rules and conventions, her ethical actions are **objectively** purposeless. They are ritualistic. The final value of her ethical system is "what a professional is supposed to do." This is not the same thing as the life, health, and well-being of her patient.

To pursue the well-being of a patient is to act purposefully. This is what the profession is all about. A nursing ethic ought to be all about what nursing and human life are all about.

LIFE AS THE FINAL VALUE

Life is the entire state of a living being. As an element of human autonomy, it is the state of a person that he experiences as his self in his world.

A sense of the value of oneself and one's life is implicit in every act of valuing. In this sense, life is a "preconscious" standard of judgment. One does not reason or analyze to one's awareness of the value of one's life. Whether well or poorly understood, one begins one's thought, analysis, and action *from* this primordial awareness.

In the health care setting, if judgment and choice are to be determined by reference to the rights and values of a patient, then the question of the central term of the nurse/patient agreement is not problematic. The central term is the patient's life and well-being.

Consider this:

- Life is the precondition of all of a patient's other values.
- Life is the precondition of a patient's rights. To respect a patient's right to autonomy, freedom, etc., and not to be concerned for his life and well-being, is, very much, to miss the point. At the same time, to be concerned with a patient's life and well-being, and not to respect his right to autonomy, freedom, etc., is to have lost one's ethical direction.
- Life is the purpose of the patient in entering the health care environment. A patient's concern for his life must be shared by his nurse, or there is no easily understood reason for her being his nurse. Life is the central term of the agreement that a nurse makes with her patient.
- A patient's motivation in entering the health care environment is the fact that his capacities and potentialities are radically circumscribed. When a patient regains his capacities and potentialities, his life is very much expanded.
- A patient, except in the most extreme circumstances, can have no rational desire before his desire to live. However, in extreme circumstances, a desire for death is not an irrational desire. It arises from a recognition of the nature of life.

Ronnie is a 7-year-old child who is dying. He comes in every week for a transfusion. One day, he says to Leah, his nurse, "I don't want this anymore." Leah explains what will happen if he does not get the transfusion. Ronnie says that he knows and he still does not want the transfusion. Leah gets the parents, physician, and other consultants together and tells Ronnie's story. Ronnie takes control of his life with Leah's help. (Woods, 1999, p. 428)

THE ROLE OF PURPOSE

It is possible to make ethical decisions with an individual person, either oneself or one's beneficiary, serving as the reference point of ethical analysis. A person does this when he or she makes human purposes the center of his or her ethical system.

There are few consistent followers of either a ritualistic or a purposive ethical system. Most people haphazardly form the ethical system they adopt. They form it out of a combination of what they have been taught by Aunt Maude or Uncle Jeffrey and their observations of effective ethical action in real life.

Ethics arose from the necessity of making decisions in the face of adversity.

A person can observe what succeeds and what fails early in life from the experiences of the everydayness of family living, the give and take of playing with playmates, and the demands of school work. A person can observe this but not everyone does.

Amy, a nurse on a cardiac step-down unit, is a case in point. Her ethical system is much more influenced by the ethical instruction force-fed to her by her Aunt Maude and Uncle Jeffrey than it is by her experience of successful and failing human interactions.

Her actions are much more ritualistic than purposive. Her actions have more in common with singing a song or reciting a poem, than with cooking a meal or mowing the lawn. The goal of singing a song or reciting a poem is simply the activity itself and nothing beyond it. The goal of cooking a meal is the finished meal. The goal of mowing a lawn is having an attractive lawn. Amy's ethical actions have no purpose beyond the actions themselves. Her ethical actions, like singing and reciting, are their own reason for being.

In the context of a person's everyday life, there is certainly nothing wrong with singing a song or reciting a poem. These can be enjoyable activities. But nonpurposive activity is very inappropriate to a bioethical context.

A purposive ethic (an ethic in the Aristotelian tradition) is one that holds, along with Aristotle and Aristoteleans, that a human person is a unitary being—that there is no moral opposition between a person's consciousness and the physical body. Modern biomedicine is much more Aristotelian than Cartesian. This is because human nature and its best potential is much more Aristotelian than Cartesian.

The Aristotelian, life-centered ethic has been under attack ever since the time of Descartes, and especially since the systematic deontology of the German philosopher Immanuel Kant (1724–1804). Since Kant, formalism and ritualism have been elevated into a worldview.

A ritualistic ethic is one that, implicitly or explicitly, holds that:

- Ethical principles are what they are apart from the desires, choices, and purposes of ethical agents.
- The reason for being of an ethical principle is to direct an ethical agent in the control of innate evil impulses.
- The desires, choices, and purposes of ethical agents are either ethically irrelevant or ethically undesirable.
- Agreement and interaction are unnecessary to ethical actions.

In the case of bioethics, a traditionalist, by the logic of his or her position, must hold that ethics is prior to, and of greater importance than, the biomedical context. The traditionalist will hold, consequently, that ethics should shape the biomedical context.

PURPOSE AS THE BASIS OF THE
BIOETHICAL STANDARDS

Purpose is the mental set of a desiring being. It also describes action directed
toward vital concerns, needs, and values. Finally, purpose signifies the needs and
values that an agent's actions are directed toward. Purpose is the central element
of a practice-based ethic. In any action that a person takes, success or failure
depends upon whether the person accomplishes his or her purpose. In an ethical
context, whether an aspect of the context is good or evil depends upon whether
it assists or hinders the purposeful actions that are called for in the context. The
intentional quality of the action is determined by the purpose—the object of the
action. An ethical action is defined in terms of its purpose.

The practical quality of an action is determined by its appropriateness to the
achievement of its purpose. In this, actions are like instruments. On the simplest
possible level, it is quite obvious that a screwdriver is right for the purpose of
screwing a screw into a piece of wood. It is wrong for the purpose of hammering
a nail. A hammer is right for hammering a nail, but wrong for screwing a screw.

A person's actions always include the mental set—the intention that inspires
the action. Intentions always include the object of the action—the goal for which
the action is intended.

If a person's purpose is to gain happiness, then those actions that will bring
about conditions that produce happiness are right and good. Those actions that
bring about conditions that undermine happiness are wrong and harmful. The
alternative is the agreement or the disagreement between context, actions, and
their purpose.

For purposes of returning a patient to a state of agency, those actions that bring
about the physical and psychological conditions of agency in a patient are right
and good. Those actions that undercut the physical or psychological conditions
of his agency are wrong and harmful.

David is in the hospital with peripheral vascular disease. His nurse, Joy, is
educating him on how he must care for himself when he leaves the hospital.

In order to do this, Joy:

- Tries to find out all she can about David so she can advise him according
  to his specific situation;
- Gives him all the information he needs so that he can enjoy the maximum
  freedom of action;
- Tells him whatever he needs to know in order to enable him to gain and
  retain his power of agency. She tells him nothing that he does not need to know
  or that might hinder his gaining and retaining his power of purposeful action;
- Allows David the isolation he needs in order to make autonomous decisions; and

• Does whatever she can in order to promote David's welfare. She does nothing that might hinder David's welfare, nothing that might hinder his power to take autonomous actions.

THE FACETS OF PURPOSE

The standard of any action, including ethical actions, is the purpose that the agent means to accomplish by the action.

Question: "Why did the chicken cross the road?"

Answer: "To get to the other side."

If a chicken, or a person, wants to walk across the road, then getting to the other side is the standard of success. If a person wants to learn to use a computer, then his or her standard of success is the ability to use a computer. If a student wants to learn to fly, then the standard of success is being able to take off, stay up, and land. If a nurse wants to recognize the self-assertion of her patient, then that patient acting on his self-assertion, or herself acting for him, is the standard of the nurse's success.

Every event that fulfills an agent's purpose is an event that signals the success of an ethical agent. The reason for being of ethical decision making is to guide the action of an ethical agent to realize such events.

The world presents various alternatives to an ethical agent. An agent chooses from among alternatives according to his or her desires. When an agent chooses from among alternatives, this act of choice forms a purposeful frame of mind. A purpose is the object of a desire that a person brings to the forefront, and retains, in his or her attention.

A choice is an objective relationship between a state of desire and a possibility that a person perceives in the world. A choice is a mental action that inspires physical action. All action is purposeful behavior.

Any purposeful ethic involves choice. An ethical system not based on purpose and choice is ritualistic and formalistic. It is like reading poetry to oneself. A ritualistic or formalistic ethic cannot motivate actions appropriate to nursing. It cannot guide a nurse's actions appropriately. It cannot enable her to objectively justify the actions she takes. It can no more be a professional ethic than tea leaf reading can be a technology.

A nurse armed with a formalistic ethic would not know what questions to ask of a context. Nor would she know what would constitute the answer to a contextual ethical question. A process of ethical justification has to do with these questions and answers. Such a process is simply an explanation of the questions a person has asked and the answers upon which she has acted.

REASON AND PURPOSE AS THE FOUNDATION
FOR ETHICAL DECISION MAKING

Purpose as an element of autonomy, in and of itself, is of primary importance in resolving an ethical dilemma. Each of the other elements of autonomy is important only as it relates to purpose.

In order to act purposefully and ethically, a nurse must always act according to the evidence she has of the array of values held by a patient. Let us examine this process through a thought experiment:

Suppose a nurse, Sylvia, stranded on a deserted island, had to make an ethical decision concerning a stranger who washed up on shore. The stranger is both naked and comatose. He has a traumatic wound to the head. Sylvia has no way of discovering the name of the stranger, let alone his specific desires, purposes, or values. Nonetheless, it is quite possible for Sylvia's action in regard to this stranger to be determined according to a proper nursing ethic. In this situation, she can use the element of purpose to arrive at perfectly justifiable decisions and actions.

Every nurse, in every situation of this type, with little difficulty, can come up with an answer to these interrelated questions:

- What would the maximum number of persons most desire in this circumstance?
- What would be the purpose of the maximum number of persons in this circumstance if they could act for themselves?

Any decision that a nurse would make on the basis of a reasoned answer to these questions is ethically justifiable. There would, in fact, be no other ethically justifiable way of arriving at a decision. If a health care professional has virtually no evidence to go on, he or she must go on what little evidence is available. This is how decisions should be made for those who cannot participate and for whom we have no prior knowledge of what they would want.

Sylvia has evidence of the sex and approximate age of the stranger. This tells her almost nothing. She can see that the stranger is human. This tells her all that she needs to know.

It is perfectly reasonable for Sylvia to form her conclusion according to the purposes that most persons would hold. Whatever purposes the maximum number of persons would hold in this circumstance, this stranger would **probably** hold. When **probability** is all you have, then you must act on the basis of what you have.

A fireman leaving a burning house might see a packet of letters and a scrapbook on a table. If he can only save one, he has a perplexing problem. He has no way of knowing which the homeowners would prefer he save. Sylvia has no such problem.

Suppose that the stranger in our thought experiment were conscious. Sylvia can see that he is bleeding from the cut on his head. Under these circumstances, Sylvia would probably act automatically and without stopping to ask permission. But Sylvia might ask him if he wants her to stop the bleeding. The odds are overwhelming that the stranger would reply that he did. Then she would know exactly what the context requires.

Sylvia does not have all this evidence. She does, however, have all the evidence that she needs. She has enough evidence on which to make a reasoned judgment. **In a circumstance of this type, the fact that it is reasoned is sufficient to justify the judgment.**

In an emergency, a health care professional will almost automatically act for the purpose of saving lives. What other justification could the health care professional have for this except that the maximum number of people in the maximum number of circumstances would want their lives to be saved? Sylvia is justified by the fact that any individual person in the emergency would almost certainly want to be saved.

It is not necessary to be a tarot card reader to be an effective ethical agent.

That she will act according to her best judgment forms part of a nurse's implicit agreement with her patient. It forms part of her relationship to the rest of the world. It is a fundamental part of her role.

However, some people are very strange.

Suppose that the stranger for whom Sylvia acted were to claim that the decision she made was a wrong decision. Suppose, for want of a better supposition, that he believes that a woman touching his head on a Tuesday defiles him. He declares that he would have preferred bleeding to death to being defiled.

Let us examine the implications of this:

Under the circumstances, Sylvia made her decision on the basis of all the evidence available to her—the evidence she had of the stranger being a person.

If the decision she made and the action she took, based on her analysis of the evidence, were a wrong decision and action, then either:

A. It is a fact that the majority of people washed onto the shore of a desert island, with scalp lacerations, would want to bleed to death and Sylvia should have known this,

or

B. Sylvia made a mistake when she reasoned from the evidence that was presented to her. An ethical agent should not make decisions by reasoning from evidence.

If the stranger attempts to justify his claim on alternative **A**, he attempts to justify it on an absurdity. Imagine a group of people with profusely bleeding scalp wounds sitting on a beach and replying to offers of help with, "No thanks, don't bother. I would just as soon bleed to death." Try to imagine this.

If the stranger attempts to justify his claim by alternative **B**, that Sylvia ought not to have acted on a reasoned conclusion based on her evidence, then his position is even more absurd.

If she ought not to have decided according to her recognition of the evidence, then she ought to have acted without thinking. But, if she ought to have acted without thinking, then anything she did would be right. If a person ought to act without thinking, then there is no way that what she does can be wrong. In this case, his claim that she should not to have taken the actions she did contradicts itself.

Let us assume that Sylvia ought to have decided on what to do without thinking, without reasoning according to the evidence available to her. If a person's action is based on thinking then, within limits, that action will be predictable. Thinking will limit the number of actions that might be taken. If a person acts without thinking, then her ensuing action will be unpredictable. There will be nothing to limit the number of actions that might be taken.

If Sylvia ought to have acted without thinking, she might have done anything at all. If she would have been right to do anything at all, then any action she took would be justified. If any action she took would be justified, then the decision and action that she actually did take could not rationally be condemned.

In the nature of things, a nurse can justify her ethical decisions and actions through the element of purpose. Purpose is, or ought to be, directly or indirectly, the standard of, just as it is the motivation of, all ethical decision making.

Every person is unique, but every person is a unique **person** and, in being a person, is the same as every other person and ethically equal to every other person. Sometimes, as in this case, a decision must be made on the basis of a person's "**sameness**." Every human being, and his every virtue, is purposive. It is always safe to assume that if what you are dealing with is a human being, then what you are dealing with has purposes. This, in itself, when necessary, justifies ethical action.

Dilemma 10-6   Jody Smith, a retired nurse, with three adult children and numerous adult grandchildren, lives in a small rural area on a limited income. Two months ago, she fell and broke her left hip. After surgery for an artificial hip replacement, she was transferred to a rehabilitation center where she had a left-side cerebrovascular accident (CVA). Upon her readmittance to the acute care facilities, she received aggressive therapy for the CVA.

Completely paralyzed on her left side, Mrs. Smith has decided that she no longer desires aggressive therapy and frequently asks the staff why she cannot die in peace. "The rehabilitation is so painful and I'll never walk again. What's the use?"

Both the physicians and her family are much more optimistic. The orthopedic surgeon is convinced that she will walk again, and the neurologist believes that she will make a full recovery and be able to return home and care for herself. Both physicians have excluded Mrs. Smith from their conversations, assuring her children that she will be "as good as new." And ignoring her request to discontinue anticoagulants and rehabilitative therapy.

Mrs. Smith refuses to cooperate with the physical and occupational therapists, will not take her medications, and refuses to perform simple tasks, relying instead on staff members to meet her activities of daily living. What should be done? (Guido, 1997).

THE ROLE OF AGENCY

The Nature of Ethical Action

Imagine, if you will, that you are taking a stroll over a very large lawn by a wood side. As you walk, you pass one by one, a rock, a tree, and then a horse. Finally, you pass a young woman and a young man.

From the viewpoint of the rock, nothing is either good or evil. Whatever happens, it is a matter of perfect indifference. But in order to experience the ethical aspects of what you see during your stroll, imagine that one thing, if only this one thing, is good in relation to the rock. There is a very weak sense in which the (only) good for the rock is to retain its structural integrity, to retain its "rockhood." Obviously, the rock is not conscious of a desire to remain in existence. That is not important. What is important is this: There is nothing morally outrageous in the fact that the rock exists and remains in existence.

Now you pass a tree. This is a very different kind of thing. The rock is inert and inanimate; the tree is alive. To stay alive, the tree must sink its roots into the earth in order to draw stability and sustenance from the ground. So you encounter a sort of progression, a change in the way of being. Even so, there is nothing here, in the living and acting of the tree, that is morally undesirable. Life is not, in itself, an ethical disaster.

Now you come to the horse. The horse is also alive. It is alive in an even stronger sense than the tree. The horse is conscious of its environment. It moves about from place to place in a manner that follows from its nature. The horse eats grass from the ground and apples from the tree. Yet, even in this behavior of the horse, there is no basis for a rational moral indignation. The existence of the horse is not a moral calamity.

So it is also with the man and woman. Here again one comes to a different kind of being—the man and woman are not only conscious, they are conscious on an abstract and conceptual level. Yet there is nothing anymore intrinsically immoral in the existence of reason in the man and woman than there is in the animality of the horse. There is nothing more morally undesirable in the animality of the horse than there is in the treeness of the tree. There is nothing more morally undesirable in the treeness of the tree than there is in the rockness of the rock.

In a nursing context, an ethical system that would seek to work around the "disaster" of a patient's being human and being alive would be a tragic mistake. It would be the opposite of an intelligible, practice-based system.

ACTION

The term "action" in ethics has a very specific and technical meaning. It can be most easily understood in relation to its correlative, "passion." Action and passion are both forms of behavior.

A passion is any behavior that an entity undergoes through a force external to itself and not as an outcome of any act of self-determination. An action is a behavior that an agent initiates. The agent determines the execution of the action, the occurrence and the nature of the behavior. Scratching an intolerable itch or behavior exhibited under the influence of an overwhelming emotion, such as fear, are instances of passion. The falling of a leaf, the careening of a billiard ball, the behavior of a nail in the vicinity of a magnet are also examples of passion.

Making and completing long-range plans, meeting an inconvenient ethical responsibility, engaging in a difficult, unfamiliar thought process, and lifting a heavy weight are various types of action. These, of course, are things that leaves, billiard balls, and nails cannot do.

In relation to a force that precludes volitional choice and compels behavior, a (potential) agent is "passive." This meaning of the term passive is retained in the adjective and in the noun "patient"; indeed, both terms have the same root. A patient is a person who is passive—a person who is incapable of actions according to normal capabilities.

Action, on the other hand, involves these preconditions:

1. An agent's awareness of the situation in which he is to act;
2. An agent's awareness of himself in general, plus his specific awareness of himself in relation to the situation in which he is to act;
3. An agent's implicit awareness of his capacity for self-determined behavior. All these capabilities can be possessed by a patient. What the patient lacks, to a greater or lesser extent, is the fourth capability.

4. The capability to translate his awareness into an action intended to bring about a desired result.

These preconditions of agency belong to every agent and are not inherently problematic. However, these potential assets of an agent can become problematic under the influence of a dilemma, when an agent may forget possession of these abilities, distort his or her relationship to them, or be unable to estimate what he or she can accomplish through them.

A nurse may find the physical or mental condition of her patient's functioning as a kind of dilemma, causing him to lose his awareness of, or even his interest in, his powers of agency. The demands of effective nursing, under these circumstances, call upon a nurse to rekindle this awareness if possible. This requires that she recognize the difference between her patient's passive acceptance of various circumstances and his actual exercise of agency. An action actually expresses the nature and intention of the agent, whereas passive acceptance may not.

AGENCY AS THE BASIS OF THE BIOETHICAL STANDARDS

A person's agency is the power to act on autonomous desires that spring from his or her own reasoning. Agency is what human life is all about.

Agency requires autonomous desire.[1] Without autonomous desire, behavior is involuntary. Involuntary behavior does not arise from agency. For instance, if a person is jostled in the street and bumps into a wall, that behavior does not arise from agency. His behavior, as we have discussed, is a passion—it arises from a force outside of his agency.

Agency requires reason or autonomous thought. Behaviors that arise entirely from the emotions, as well as reflex behaviors, are not actions. Actions express the specific nature of the agent who acts. Only rational beings possess agency. Only reason in action expresses the specific nature of a rational being.

If ethical action does not, in fact, properly begin with attention to agency, with actions that arise in a patient's autonomous desire and reason, then all of bioethics is misdirected. The health care setting is designed to promote the regaining of agency in the service of a patient's individual purposes. For this reason, every bioethical standard has the same purpose.

- The standard of autonomy is designed to protect those actions of a patient that express his unique character-structure.
- The standard of freedom is designed to protect actions arising from the individual agency of the patient.

- The standard of objectivity is designed to support the actions that arise from the individual agency of a patient. It does this by allowing him to act on his own knowledge and awareness.
- The standard of self-assertion is designed to protect the self-ownership of a patient insofar as that self-ownership is expressed in the patient's self-initiated actions.
- The standard of beneficence is designed to protect the actions of an agent—to support his actions and to see that no harm comes to his power of agency.
- The standard of fidelity is designed to protect his objective attention to his self-interest and to the values he pursues, as well as to protect a person's self-awareness of the interactions of several agents as they act toward interwoven purposes.

Try to imagine applying the bioethical standards to a machine and you will see the essential relationship between the standards and the patient's agency.

AGENCY, RIGHTS,[2] AND ETHICAL INTERACTION

Imagine a desert island with only one inhabitant, Jane. With no possibility of a division of labor, and none of the tools of civilization available to her, survival is a pressing problem for Jane. Under these circumstances, what does Jane have a right to do and what does she have no right to do—what would it be wrong for her to do?

In these highly unusual circumstances, it is obvious that Jane has the right to do whatever she has the power to do. Her right to take action is unlimited.

She has the right to pursue any value that she has reason to believe will bring her benefit and the right to shun whatever would tend to her detriment. She has as much right to pursue her values as she has to exist—and each for the same reason.

How could it be wrong for Jane to act to sustain her life? Why would it be wrong for her to act toward the realization of her values? There is no logical reason why Jane should negate any aspect of her being, neither the fact **that** she is nor the fact of **what** she is.

The fact that Jane, a thinking, valuing person, actually exists is exhaustive evidence that it is right that she should exist. The fact that Jane is, by nature, a being to whom the pursuit of values is appropriate is conclusive evidence that it is right that she pursue that which she values. Against the fact that Jane does exist, no rational evidence can be adduced to show that it would be ethically better if she did not exist. The proposition that Jane ought to renounce her life or the pursuit of her values cannot be logically or, therefore, ethically justified. It simply does not make sense.

Jane has the right to be what she is. Any alternative to this principle is incoherent. As a natural corollary to this principle, we must conclude that Jane has a right to do whatever she has the power to do. Nothing Jane does can violate the rights of another. There is no other on the island.

Now, let us change the scenario somewhat.

One day, Michelle is washed ashore. Holding strictly to the context of our problem, how has Jane's situation changed? How is the principle that Jane has the right to do whatever she has the power to do been modified?

Ethically, the principle is unimpaired, although two significant changes have come into Jane's life:

1. As rational beings, Michelle and Jane have an obligation not to violate each other's rights. Whether they do violate each other rights, the obligation remains. The obligation is there, not by virtue of any arbitrary decision either might make, but by virtue of their defining characteristics, by virtue of what Jane and Michelle have in common—their rational nature. As a corollary of this, each has an obligation to honor the agreements that she makes with the other.

2. Jane's existential position is enormously enhanced, as is Michelle's for having found Jane there.

> There are many things outside us which are useful to us and which, therefore, are to be sought. Of all these, none more excellent can be discovered than those that exactly agree with our nature. If, for example, two individuals of exactly the same nature are joined together, they make up a single individual, doubly stronger than each alone. Nothing, therefore, is more useful to man than man. (Spinoza, 1949, pp. 202–203)

If the inhabitants of the island number two or number in the millions, nothing is essentially changed. Moreover, allow yourself a little thought experiment by placing yourself in the picture. If you were Michelle or Jane, the ethical principles governing the situation would remain exactly the same. You lack no right that others possess. You possess no right that others lack.

If any ethical circumstance that might apply to a particular individual is, all things being equal, right or wrong, it can only be because it is right or wrong universally, for every ethical agent.

THE BIOLOGICAL FUNCTION OF AGENCY

Agency is the agent's interaction with his own life. It is the instrument of reason and desire. It is the servant of an agent's purpose.

The function of purpose is to move an agent from a lesser to a greater level of autonomy, freedom, objective connection to reality, self-ownership, power to pursue values, and fidelity to his life. The function of agency is to move an agent from a less refined reason and a less complete knowledge to a more refined reason and a more complete knowledge. It guides reason in its vision of rational desires and in actions leading to the fulfillment of desire. It enables an agent to attain a more desirable condition of being.

Finally, agency serves to increase its own competency and strength. In taking physical actions, a person increases the strength of her body. In taking the actions necessary to increase understanding, a person increases the strength of her mind.

AGENCY AND RIGHTS

In the life of every (noncriminal) individual and in the history of humanity, it becomes evident that the range and effectiveness of the individual person's activities are greatly augmented if people do not have to devote time and effort to guarding themselves against aggression, coercion, and fraud. So, as a sort of evolutionary instrument, an implicit agreement arises among rational beings, an agreement not to aggress against, not to coerce, and not to defraud each other.

It is also the essential basis of the existence of laws. Laws arise because there is a need for them. But the need arose long before the laws. This implicit agreement arose before the laws were possible. It arose with the human ability to make agreements.

Before any laws were ever made, the necessary relations of justice existed. "To say that nothing is just or unjust except that which is commanded or forbidden by positive law is as absurd as saying that before a circle is actually drawn its radii are not equal" (De Montesquieu, 1949, p. 108).

To the extent that a society is free, the laws that it recognizes as most fundamental are reflections of individual rights. These laws are an explicit statement of the implicit agreement on nonaggression.

Where laws have no rational justification, where they serve no evident need, and where they have no moral basis, they are resented and notoriously difficult to enforce. Not so with laws based on the implicit agreement—perhaps not even a criminal can resent such laws.

This preexisting agreement against aggression arises from the human condition. Without it, there would be no basis for honoring any inconvenient explicit agreements. No legal system could possibly be effective. There would be no basis for agreement on a legal system. The only check on people's criminality would be the limits of their imaginations and the range of their daring.

Making an agreement is not at all synonymous with having reason to believe that an agreement will be kept. Where there is no positive reason to believe that an agreement will be kept, there is no practical reason to make an agreement. Dependable, explicit agreements are made possible by this implicit agreement.

We have defined **rights** as being: The product of an implicit agreement among rational beings, by virtue of their rationality, not to obtain actions nor the product of actions from others except through voluntary consent objectively gained. This implicit agreement gives fiber to explicit agreements and to laws. It gives moral force to every explicit agreement and every other implicit agreement. This holds true of the unspoken agreement between nurse and patient. The nurse/patient agreement is, in effect, guaranteed by the implicit agreement that constitutes rights. It is an agreement that nurse and patient have a right to expect that each will fulfill his or her role according to the purposes that motivate their interaction. It is an agreement that there will be fidelity and benevolence on each side.

The English philosopher, John Stuart Mill (1806–1873), said that one person cannot advance the interests of another by compulsion. One person cannot rightly compel another person to do something because it is better for that other person to do it, because it will make the other person happier, or because, in the opinion of the first person, it would be wise for the second person to do it (1988).

Rights determine the actions an agent can take. Everyone has the right to be free from the coercion of others. Everyone constantly relies on the species-wide agreement that people will not deal with each other coercively. A person can act freely in any social context as long as he or she does not coerce another. In coercing another, a person gives up the right to exercise freedom. It is well said that:

> [The right to] self determination is an individual's exercise of the capacity to form, revise, and pursue personal plans for life . . . free from outside control. . . . In the context of health care, self determination overrides practitioner determination. (President's Commission, 1982, p. 32)

A nurse, because she is the agent of her patient, and through the implicit agreement she has with him, has agreed to protect the rights of her patient. She has an ethical obligation to protect her patient from anyone who would violate his rights. Above all, she cannot, herself, break the rights agreement.

It has been observed that rights is to a society what reason is to an individual. The health care setting is a small society.

Dilemma 10-7   Jason is a patient in a psychiatric hospital. He was admitted nonvoluntarily. He has been diagnosed as a paranoid schizophrenic. His physician has prescribed 5 mg Haldol and 2 mg Cogentin. Jason refuses to take the medication. He tells his nurse, Jessica, that the physician is trying to poison him. Aside from what he tells her, Jessica has no reason to believe that Jason's physician is trying to poison him. Would she be justified in giving Jason an injection of the medication against his will so that he would get the benefit of it? Would doing so violate Jason's rights?

MUSINGS

A knowledge of the bioethical standards is an essential part of a nurse's context of knowledge. However, it is possible to go beyond the bioethical standards.

As we have seen, the individual standards can **appear** to come into conflict. There can also be a conflict in the **interpretation** of an individual standard. It is desirable that there be a way to resolve these conflicts. That way is a knowledge of the ethical elements—the elements of human autonomy.

No one can be human and be completely unfamiliar with that which makes him or her autonomous. Everyone is familiar with the elements of human autonomy, at least, on an implicit level. It is quite advantageous for a professional to become familiar with them explicitly.

To interact on a human level is to interact on a highly intimate level. People interact with each other on an intimate level when they understand each other's desires. Desire is the basis of meaning and purpose in every human life. Intimacy rests on meaning and purpose.

The highest advantage of a patient is his professional's desire to be a professional. The appropriate ethical focus of a professional is the desire of her patient. Her patient's desire is final. But, in any context, only his reason can validate his desires.

The interweaving of their desires is the ethical basis for the nurse/patient agreement. This agreement is seldom, and probably never, verbalized. It is an implicit agreement arising immediately between them. The ultimate basis of this agreement, therefore, is not anything the nurse or the patient says. It is what they **are** that determines what they ought to do.

A professional's exercise of reason is her greatest source of ethical confidence and strength. As the agent of her patient, confidence and strength are values that she offers him and herself. She owes it to herself to exercise reason in developing the virtues that her profession requires.

In every case, the benefits that accrue to the patient logically imply the benefits that accrue to the professional. Their interaction ought to enhance both of their lives. This is the place for a concern for life to begin.

There is one activity more central to human life than any other. This is the discovery and pursuit of autonomous purposes. It is the activity that relates an individual's abstract aspirations and the biological functions necessary to the organism's continued survival.

An individual person defines what is important and what is not by the purposes he or she chooses to pursue. This is the basis of a purposive, practice-based ethic.

Every action in a bioethical context is taken for a purpose. This purpose taken in a bioethical context is some biomedical good. This good is specific to the welfare of one or more individual patients.

If any action in any ethical system is not well intentioned, then it is not justifiable. Every action, in any ethical context, is taken with a view to good or evil. In a practice-based ethical system, the effects of an action are fully as important as the intention behind the action. The quality of the ethical action, which is to say, whether it is good or evil, is determined by the intention behind it **and** by its predictable effects.

Figure 10.1 includes the elements of autonomy.

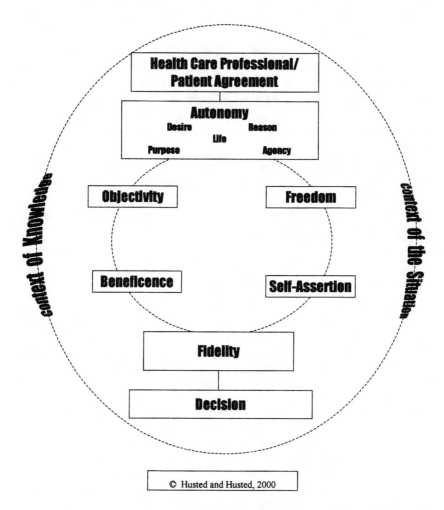

FIGURE 10.1 Husteds' symphonological bioethical decision-making advanced guide.

NOTES

1. We define desire as including, "all of the physiological and psychological processes that constitute the life of an individual person."

This gives the concept of desire an organic grounding. Without this organic grounding, human desire may easily seem to be either arbitrary—whimsical, transient, and, therefore, unimportant, or a passion—a behavior entirely determined from outside the organism. This would make it of no greater ethical value than any other externally determined passion. But desire is an expression of the essential being of a human individual.

Given an organic, vis a vis, a purely psychological grounding, it follows that, e.g., a tree in the actions of its roots and leaves exhibits a form of desire. In man, the same kind of organic actions occur, but man is aware of these actions and the accompanying circumstances of his organism. It is this awareness that is referred to as desire. But desire includes these conditions and actions of the organism of which man is conscious. All of these constitute the desire of the living being.

2. Strictly speaking, rights only exists in situations where more than one person is involved. A right is a right against another person—a right not to be aggressed against. So when we speak of "one's rights on a desert island," we are using the term rights in an extended sense to refer to what would be equivalent to rights among a number of people.

REFERENCES

De Montesquieu, S. (1949). *Spirit of the laws* (T. Nuggent, Trans.). New York: Random House. (Original work published 1748)

Guido, G. W. (1997). *Legal issues in nursing* (2nd ed.). Stamford, CT: Appleton & Lange.

Husted, J. H. (1987). Spinoza's conception of the attributes of substance. *The Metaphysics of Substance: The Proceedings of the American Catholic Philosophical Association, LXI,* 121–131.

Mill, J. S. (1988). *On liberty.* New York: Penguin. (Original work published 1819)

Milstead, J. A. (1999). Advanced practice nurses and public policy, naturally. In J. A. Milstead (Ed.), *Health policy and politics* (pp. 1–41). Gaithersburg, MA: Aspen.

President's Commission for the Study of Ethical Problems and Medicine and Biomedical and Behavioral Research. (1982). *Making health care decisions: The ethical and legal implication of informed consent in the patient-practitioner relationship.* (Vol. 1). Washington, DC: U.S. Government Printing Office.

Rasmussen, D. B., & Den Uyl, D. J. (1991). *Liberty and nature: An Aristotelian defense of liberal order.* LaSalle, IL: Open Court.

Spinoza, B. (1949). *Ethics*. (J. Gutmann, Ed.). New York: Hafner Publishing. (Original work published 1675)

Woods, M. (1999). A nursing ethic: The moral voice of experienced nurses. *Nursing Ethics, 6*, 423–433.

CHAPTER 11

Advanced Concepts in Symphonological Theory

"I am a man, nothing human is alien to me." (Terence, 163 B.C.)

W e all live in the same world. Our life is made possible by agreements. We all have the same world to understand and a human way of understanding it. We are all faced with the need to act to achieve happiness—a state of success with ourselves, and to avoid unhappiness—a sense of ourselves failing as humans. This involves the need to make decisions. Ethics is the art of making these decisions.

Every person has a philosophy of life, whether or not the person realizes it. This philosophy impacts on the person's professional philosophy and guides approaches she takes to her role as a health care professional (Gaberson & Oermann, 1999).

Symphonology is a bioethical theory. In being a bioethical theory, it clarifies the purposes of a profession. The essential aspects of nursing and health care have to do with the ethical practice of the health care professional and her relationship to her patient. A nursing and health care theory is one that should direct its practitioners to appropriate ways of practicing.

METAPHYSICS

The universe we live in is structured in such a way that the processes that existents act or interact to produce on a broad, even infinite, scale are replicated on very small scales. The Aristotlean tradition pointed out a fact on which all of our experience and our belief in the order of the universe is based. This is the fact that the characteristic action of every existent arises from the nature of the existent. In consequence of this, the characteristic interaction of several existents follows on their natures in relation to each other. These different sorts of processes are sufficiently similar, in their form and functioning, to justify inclusion under one, highly abstract, concept—the concept of "agreement."

The concept of agreement signifies, on every level, **a propensity or formal potentiality in existents to behave in specific ways and no others when they are interacting, based on the nature of each existent**. On each level, agreement consists in their interacting in a form necessary to that level.

The agreement between existents is a relationship between their natures, arising by virtue of their formal structure and producing specific interactions through offers and acceptances characterizing that level of existence. The levels of agreement particularly relevant to symphonology are the:

Natural Agreement—An agreement among things that they will interact according to the nature of each.[1] For instance, a leaf will be carried by the wind. The nature of the wind is such that it has a propensity to carry light objects such as leaves. The nature of a leaf is such that it will 'allow itself' to be carried by wind.

Natural agreements arise through the nature of each existent. Their natures produce intelligible and predictable interactions. Natural agreement is the objective foundation of purpose in purposive beings. A purpose always involves rearranging and redirecting things according to the possibilities afforded by natural agreements.

Instrumental Agreement—A natural agreement compatible with a purpose. It is the agreement of an instrument to serve a purpose. This type of natural agreement arises in the same way as any other natural agreement—according to the natures of the things that affect each other—but according to human or animal purposes. Specific instances of this agreement are hammer and nail, screwdriver and screw, a boat on water, bees building a hive with the material that makes this possible, and beavers using trees to build a dam.

Vital Agreement—An agreement between the life of a living thing and the organic conditions necessary to its life or survival. It is life's agreement with itself. The vital agreement is the subject matter of medical knowledge. It is the interaction of an organism with itself—a form of natural agreement based on a most fundamental level of purpose—the organic level. The vital agreement exists on the level of purpose of which conscious purpose is an outgrowth. Nonpoisonous food, climates compatible with life, abstract values to be envisioned and pursued, and the means of protection from enemies are, in effect, instruments assisting the organism in sustaining its vital agreement. The circulation of the blood and the process of respiration are some examples of the organism acting to sustain its vital agreement with itself.

Cognitive Agreement—An agreement of the understanding with the object that is understood—the agreement holding between a knowing mind and its known object. It is a propensity of consciousness in its act of being conscious. Examples of this type of agreement are a dog and master recognizing each other, grasping the existence of instrumental agreements, the awareness of temporal and spatial relations, and recognition of the meaning of words.

Ethical Agreement—An agreement between cognition and the various vital agreements—an agreement between a vital agreement as the object of knowledge and a cognitive agreement as knowledge of the nature of the vital agreement. It is a form of cognitive agreement. It functions in actions intended to serve the interests of life. Some examples are self-interest, the rights' agreement, and agreements that establish human interactions.

Formal Agreement—An agreement between agents to interact on the basis of complementary motivations. It is perfect or imperfect insofar as it involves the character-structures and virtues of interagents—those who interact. Formal agreements produce interaction based on trade and formulated in a meeting of the minds. The formal agreement is an outgrowth of cognitive agreements, and is made possible by the ability of conscious beings to achieve a meeting of the minds. A familiar example is the health care professional/ patient agreement. **The objectivity and rationality of formal agreements depend, in every instance, on their harmony with the more basic levels of agreement.**

The objectivity and rationality of a formal agreement depends on its harmony with

Natural agreements—the availability of whatever is necessary to fill the agreement.

Instrumental agreements—the ability of interagents to turn these objects into instruments for the accomplishing of the agreement.

Vital agreements—harmony between the formal agreement and the requirements of human life and flourishing.

Cognitive agreements—possession of the knowledge necessary to recognize the causal relationships that make circumstances intelligible, and foresight into probable consequences possible.

Ethical agreements—possession of knowledge of how this agreement will promote life and well being and not conflict with the purposes—the life and flourishing of the interacting agents.

In each case, agreement is a propensity of existents to behave in specific ways and no others when they are interacting—based on the nature of each existent. When one takes note of how the different levels of agreement intertwine, how each level is dependent on the "lower" levels, and how it is not possible to put concrete examples of agreement into one isolated level, the relationship of dependence between the levels of agreement becomes clear.

EPISTEMOLOGY

Knowledge

The two most plausible epistemological theories are conceptualism and moderate realism. Conceptualism is the theory that concepts are formed through the similarities of similar things; that the nature of an individual thing cannot impress itself on the mind; that the mind is not capable of discovering the nature of an isolated individual thing. Moderate realism is the theory that concepts are formed through the abstract sameness of things; that the source of human knowledge is its discovery of the nature of individual things. It presupposes that the mind is capable of discovering the nature of an individual thing. The theory most appropriate to the health care setting is moderate realism.

Conceptualists claim that one can form, e.g., the concept "round," by virtue of the fact that round things are similar in being round. Moderate realists claim that, insofar as two things are similar in being round, they are, abstractly, the same.

This certainly seems like a quibble. Much bad philosophy arises from a choice of the wrong side of a quibble.

In the health care setting, a very common, implicit, and undetected error—a mind-set—is to understand a patient in the manner of conceptualism. "This patient is sick because he has what that patient has and that patient is sick. Everyone who is similar in having this condition is sick. This is what makes him a patient." A conceptualist viewpoint brings health care professionals to understand patients through the fact that patients are similar. This implies that an individual patient can be understood in terms applicable to all patients—without being understood as an individual. Additionally, a certain course of action is ethically appropriate to this patient because it is ethically appropriate to that patient and that patient's context is similar to this patient's context.

Conceptualism is dreadfully inadequate as a theory to guide professional interaction.

Moderate realism would hold that this patient is sick because his present physiological or psychological state is inadequate to normal vital function. A moderate realist approach brings a health care professional to understand a patient through the fact that, one by one, patients are who they are. This implies that an individual patient must, and can, be understood through his unique character-structures, or a certain course of action is beneficent in relation to this patient because this course of action would best nurture and strengthen **his** character-structures.

Truth

The two most plausible theories of truth are the coherence theory and the correspondence theory. Coherence is the theory that a belief is true if it is logically coherent with the collection of one's other true beliefs. This perspective is pandemic in the health care system. It dovetails neatly with conceptualism. It is, in effect, conceptualism applied to beliefs. "This belief is true because it is coherent with (does not contradict) that belief and that belief is true." And so on into a whirlpool of subjectivism.

In the emotivism that dominates much ethical decision making in the health care setting, the process goes as follows: "This assumption must be true because it coheres (does not conflict) with my emotional state. Assumptions that cohere with my emotional state are true. More than this, they are good, right, and justifiable."

The correspondence theory holds that a belief is true when it arises from, is formed by, and "corresponds" with the state of affairs that is the object of the belief.

The alternatives, as ethical perspectives, are:

For coherence: "This dilemma arouses in me a specific set of beliefs and feelings. These beliefs and feelings do not contradict beliefs I presently hold, and do not disturb my current emotional state. Therefore, these beliefs and feelings constitute a valid judgment."

For correspondence: "Given my examination and analysis of this dilemma, I have formed the following belief that I hold to be adequate to explain its nature, and to suggest appropriate responses."

It must be obvious that an effective professional cannot make decisions appropriate to dilemmas in the health care setting based on an examination of the ideas, beliefs, and attitudes preexisting in her mind and brought to her attention by a superficial experience of the dilemma. It must be just as obvious that an effective professional must make decisions appropriate to dilemmas based on an adequate understanding of the dilemma achieved through the acquisition of beliefs correspondent with the nature of the dilemma.

A decision maker must:

Work with clues that could mean many different things,
Pay attention to clues that are important,
Ignore clues that are not important,
Integrate apparently random data into a meaningful pattern,
Work with data that cannot easily be explained,
Carry intelligence from the mind into the circumstance through "indwelling" in the circumstance,
Recognize a coherent pattern among clues,
Perform feats of integration without being aware of what he is doing,

Tacitly integrate clues into meaning, and
Move from clues or parts to wholes (Polanyi, 1974).

Only moderate realism and correspondence make this possible.

METAETHICS

Many health care professionals embrace either a traditional ethical system or a contemporary ethical fad. Many others, discouraged by these ethical outlooks, either become calloused in relation to their profession and their patients, or they, haphazardly, become benevolent. They give no explicit attention to the ethical underpinnings of their interactions. They lose concern for an understanding of what it is about their profession that makes it a worthwhile endeavor.

Is there value to the profession? Does it have meaning? Does it serve a purpose? If so, then there are alternatives. There are choices to be made. The profession can be practiced effectively or badly. The profession calls for an ethical perspective—an ethic specific to itself, a practice-based ethic.

A practice-based ethic, if it is to serve and enhance practice, must possess integrity. It must be faithful to the profession, to the professional and her patient, and faithful to itself. If it defeats its purpose, it becomes another externally related system of evasion.

A practice-based ethic must serve to keep professional and patient on intelligible, cause and effect, courses of interaction. This requires direction toward a state of affairs taken as a final cause and an objective principle of judgment. For every human profession, in one way or another, this principle is human survival and flourishing. For the health care professional, it is the life, health, and well-being of sick and disabled individuals.

There is no absolute disability without a weakness of the virtues. There is no absolute health without their strength.

Ethical agents are never more useful to one another than when each is strengthening the virtues—the power to survive and flourish—of the other. To do this is to meet the demands of justice—a causal relationship, the purpose of which is to benefit one another, enrich each other.

This is the invigorating, and mostly undiscovered, essence of nursing. Like the picture that is worth 1,000 words, demonstration is the best form of teaching. It teaches the patient. Even more so, it teaches the agent—the health care professional. It is an ancient truth that the best way to learn is to teach.

MUSINGS

The virtue of a professional, as a professional, is to recognize and accept the lower levels of agreement. The virtues of a professional, as an ethical agent, is to recognize and accept her formal agreement with her patient.

The existence of a formal agreement establishes the primary meaning of "obligation." If her formal agreement does not establish her sense of obligation to her practice, nothing will. That a health care professional has no obligation to honor her formal professional/patient agreement implies that she has no ethical obligations at all. If she has no ethical obligations at all, then the idea of a professional ethic involves a contradiction in terms.

If a health care professional believes that her rational self-interest is achieved, through the pursuit of her professional obligation, she is logically compelled to honor the ethical implications of her agreement. In this case, her agreement is not a flimsy thing. And it will support her stable ethical obligations. She is practicing, at least, a primitive form of symphonology whether or not she knows it.

NOTE

1. Hopefully, it will be understood that on this level of agreement there is no suggestion of conscious awareness motivating or accompanying interaction.

REFERENCES

Gaberson, K. B., & Oermann, M. H. (1999). *Clinical teaching strategies in nursing.* New York: Springer.
Polanyi, M. (1974). *Personal knowledge: Towards a post-critical philosophy.* Chicago: University of Chicago Press.
Terence, P. (163 B.C.). Heauton timoroumenos (the self tormentor), Act. I.

Use of Symphonology in Roles Other Than Direct Patient Care

CHAPTER 12

The Educator/Student/Patient Agreement

Barbara A. Brown

It is possible for teachers and students to interact on the basis of agreement. All that is necessary is a meeting of the minds. For this to occur, it is necessary for there to be a motivation toward a meeting of the minds.

Symphonology, as a practice-based ethic, functions well in the field of education. Teaching is an interactive endeavor that involves a professional relationship between teacher and student. "The art of teaching is the art of discovery" (Mark Van Doren in Maggio, 1997, p. 28). The art of learning can be summarized in the following: "A real education consists in drawing **the best out of yourself**" (Mohandas K. Gandhi in Maggio, 1997, p. 3). One does not have a real education unless one has drawn the best out of himself.

The agreement, in the case of learner and educator, is much more explicit than that between health care professional and patient. Each is much more aware of what their commitments and responsibilities are, except in the case of the very young. Each has responsibilities, and in the sense that the student is not incapacitated as a patient would be, the responsibilities are more equally shared than between health care professional and patient.

THE RELATIONSHIP OF THE BIOETHICAL STANDARDS TO EDUCATION

Each bioethical standard is relevant in the context of the learning environment.

Autonomy includes those generic human qualities that make one person the same as any other person. It also includes those individual aspects of a person that make him unique and unlike any other person. It is the generic human qualities that curricula are, and must be, built upon. However, the uniqueness, the individuality of learners, must always be a consideration of individual educators. It is the responsibility of educators to help the learner be successful, which often includes arranging things for the consideration of the individuality of the learner. Since the student is the center of the teacher's focus, the teacher must maintain sensitivity to the student's unique learning needs. This does not apply only to students with learning disabilities. According to Plato (1945), it is education that leads a person from the shadows of the cave to the light of reality. In the context of the learning experience, the bioethical standards are the basis of the teacher/student agreement and also the lens through which the learning experience should be viewed.

Freedom can be utilized to create and maintain a learning environment so that all may learn. The student must be given the freedom of inquiry. This idea is explicated eloquently in the works of Michael Polanyi (1974). Critical thinking, changes in attitude and values, and the putting together of patterns can only be facilitated through the creative use of appropriate strategies that the teacher has the freedom and the obligation to utilize. She should utilize them wisely.

Objectivity is realized when a teacher remembers that dogma or personal prejudices should not be taught as fact or knowledge. The teacher should maintain objectivity in regard to what is being taught and give the student a broad, rather than a narrow, perspective. What is taught should help the student move toward positive outcomes for his future.

Self-assertiveness, the right to control one's time and effort, encompasses both the teacher and the student. For instance, a teacher is responsible for creating assignments that are worth the time and effort necessary to accomplish the task. There must be a balance between time, effort, and learning. The educator must maintain a balance of obligations to teaching, as well as other endeavors, that enables her to do her job and to do it well. The teacher is responsible for creating an environment in the classroom, clinical, laboratory, or playground, that protects the student from intrusive contact from others who would interfere with that person's learning. This means that discipline must be maintained, albeit, benevolent discipline. Discipline should not be the central objective of a teacher's actions.

Beneficence is embodied in the concept that whatever is taught should be taught in such a way that the student will be enriched by the learning. Learning must benefit the knower. The learner must be able to relate what is learned to his experience of the world. Just as with health care, the learner is the beneficiary. (However, in clinical learning experiences, the patient must still be the focus of the student and educator's concern. The education of the student cannot take precedence over the safety and competent care of the patient.) The learner should leave the experience better off than when the educational endeavor began. This same outcome must accrue to the patient—the patient must be better off for having given the student the opportunity to learn.

Fidelity in the teacher/student agreement requires that the teacher facilitate the learning in a nonthreatening way—a way that stimulates creativity and discovery, rather than fear and stagnation. On the other hand, the learner is responsible to do whatever is necessary to learn—this requires active participation.

CONCLUSION

Behind the teacher/student agreement must always remain the agreement that both have with patients. The patient must still be central in the process.

Learning should be, can be, and ought to be pleasurable. Teacher and student working together can make this a reality (Eble, 1988).

REFERENCES

Eble, K. (1988). *The craft of teaching* (2nd ed.). San Francisco: Jossey-Bass.

Maggio, R. (1997). *Quotations on education.* Paramus, NJ: Prentice Hall.

Plato (Trans. F. M. Cornford). (1945). *The republic of Plato.* New York: Oxford University Press.

Polanyi, M. (1974). *Personal knowledge: Towards a post-critical philosophy.* Chicago: University of Chicago Press.

CHAPTER 13

The Administrator/Health Professional/Patient Agreement

Marge Hardt and Kimberly C. Hopey

I. NATURE OF ADMINISTRATIVE DECISION MAKING IN HEALTH CARE

The administrator's role in decision making in a health care organization is to link decisions that drive high quality patient care with those that fulfill their fiduciary responsibility to the community served. The administrator is faced with ethical issues when these two responsibilities are mutually exclusive. A successful administrator needs to have a clear approach when making ethical decisions at the organizational, staff, and patient levels. Symphonology provides a comprehensive framework to guide the administrator's ethical decision making practices.

An administrator participates in decision making at many different levels in the organization. The first and broadest level of decision making is that which impacts the community at large, as well as the core financial viability of the organization. This level of decision making can have significant impact on the health care programs and services provided to the community. The second level of decisions surrounds the philosophical and practical approaches to care delivery and employee relations within the health care organization. At the third and closest level to individual patients, the administrator acts as a consultant and role model when approaching ethical dilemmas related to individual patients with clinical leaders and staff members. One example of a current/future ethical issue facing the health care administrator at all three levels of decision making is managed care. The application of symphonology to administration in the managed care environment will be discussed in more depth later in this chapter.

Ethical Decision Making in Administrative Practice

Several researchers have studied the administrator's ethical decision-making process. Sietsema and Spradley (1987) conducted a descriptive study with the intent of identifying the administrative decision-making process, as well as the resources utilized when making ethical decisions. The top five resources used for resolving ethical issues were: Administrative colleagues, personal values, nursing colleagues, the "Patient Bill of Rights," and the CEO/Board of Trustees. A theory of ethics was not one of the top resources used for resolving issues in this study, which is consistent with other studies of similar subject matter (Borawski, 1995; Camunas, 1994a; 1994b). The literature cites the lack of an established ethical decision-making process to be related to the lack of exposure of administrators to ethical theory (Chown, 1992; Wilson, 1998).

The health care administrator must bounce between the global, or macro focus, to the individual, or micro focus, many times each day. The fluid use of a decision-making guide is essential to ensure adequate consideration of each situation prior to action. The use of an appropriate ethics theory will prevent the use of rules, personal values, and cultural beliefs in place of what is appropriate, given the context of knowledge and of the situation at hand. The utility of symphonology will be discussed in the following examples as it relates to ethical decision making in the administrator's practice when addressing global, as well as individual issues.

The Use of Symphonology in Administrative Decision Making

Community Level/Strategic Decision Making

The administrators and Board of Trustees represent the health care organization, as well as the community served. There are ethical decisions that are made at this level that will impact the availability of health care, as well as guide the practice of health care professionals.

One of the primary ethical issues in today's health care environment is resource allocation. In the case of limited resources, executive level leaders must choose a methodology for the prioritization of services and programs. An example of an ethical dilemma that is faced by many patient care administrators is whether to provide expensive services to patient populations when those services will result in a loss of revenue to the organization.

Deontology or utilitarianism is often chosen as an implicit framework to be used to make these difficult decisions because the application of a single concept, such as "duty" or the "greatest good," is relatively straightforward. Unfortunately, these models are not straightforward at the point of service. If the decision is made that no patient will receive the costly service (greatest good) or that the physician and nurses have a duty to advocate not only for the patient, but also for the organization's financial position, then the health care professional's agreement with the patient may not be honored.

Instead, the use of symphonology would guide the administrator to view the individual situation in the context and to strategize for the benefit of patients and the financial stability of the institution. Questions like the following can help expand the context and move toward appropriate solutions: Are there other providers who will be paid for the service if they provide it? Are there other ways of seeking payment for the patients who may need these services, and can they be established in advance of the first patient? Approaching the situation in this manner will lead to collaboration among competitors to prevent all providers from offering the same service in a fiscally irresponsible manner. It is not essential for each hospital to meet the total needs of every patient just because of the not-for-profit status. An administrator must understand the difference between ethical behavior and heroics. Putting the financial viability of the organization at risk because of a mission statement may be heroic, but it is not necessarily the only alternative. Using symphonology helps to guide the decision-making process.

The most important consideration for the administrator after these decisions are made is that there will be physicians and other health care professionals who must continue to practice in the environment that has been established. Putting physicians and nurses in a position to deny necessary care on a case-by-case basis is unacceptable because it clearly violates the professional/patient agreement. It will also lead to burn-out at an increased rate. It is essential that first-line health care employees can form and honor the professional agreement with patients and practice in the context of the patient's situation. Here the administrator can serve as a role model at the person-to-person level, giving help and support as needed. This is facilitated when the administrator utilizes the appropriate ethical decision-making approach when dealing with individuals within strategic dilemmas and lives the ethic herself.

Organizational-Level Ethical Decision Making

The health care administrator is accountable for the development of the philosophy/vision and patient-care policies that will create the environment of practice excellence. At the same time, the administrator acts to develop policies that guide employee behavior, and advocates for employees. The use of symphonology in each of these administrative arenas will be discussed.

The philosophy/vision of an organization acts as a mechanism for the communi-cation of practitioners' and patients' beliefs related to how care should be delivered. It is the administrator's role to coordinate the articulation of this vision. Sympho-nology, utilized as a conceptual framework and decision-making tool, emphasizes the importance of viewing the professional/patient agreement within the context of the situation and assists practitioners in clarifying their role in the care and decision-making processes.

An organization's policies are tools for communicating the patient-care philoso-phy. Take for example the organization's visiting-hours policy. If symphonology is the guiding focus used in the organization, then the visiting-hours policy would be supportive of the care provider and patient making decisions related to appro-priate visitation for the individual patient. It would allow for maximal flexibility and would not be written as a one-size-fits-all policy, such as a rules-based policy. This makes the overall assumption that health care employees are able to work with patients to make decisions that foster the professional/patient agreement, and that professionals have the ability to think and act appropriately in difficult situations.

Policies or the "breaking of policies" is often a core issue in the disillusionment of practitioners. The more experienced decision maker requires an environment that promotes contextual decision making that has a direct benefit for the patient (Benner, Tanner, & Chesla, 1996). If policies are too narrow or overabundant, then the message is sent that practitioners are to "go by the book" and not enter into meaningful agreements with patients. It sends the message to remain external to the context and follow the rules. If the quality of patient care is to be truly excellent, then it is essential for the environment to support excellent decision making.

Symphonology can also be used as a framework for the development of policies that guide employee behavior. Application of the theory in the development of policies will decrease the need for its use in ethical issues down the road. As with all human resource policies, the organization strives for consistency so that all employees are treated with equal fairness. The unfortunate truth about this practice is that not all employee situations are, in fact, equal. A human resource policy needs to give the leader discretionary judgment. This enables the leader to then be able to make a decision within the context of the situation and the context of knowledge related to that particular employee. This will, at times, result in "inequity," but will be seen as superior leadership in the long run. This type of decision making requires a framework not guided by rules, but by the context and capabilities of all relevant participants.

Now we will use the example of the attendance policy of a particular organiza-tion. Suppose the organization's policy states that after five sick occurrences in a rolling year, the employee receives written discipline. Consider the nurse who has a very solid work history and good attendance for the last 10 years, however, during the last few months has had an unusual amount of sick time usage and reached five occurrences. If the policy is rule based, and the leader follows the policy, then written discipline will be administered to this employee. The employee will feel poorly treated because he/she has been a reliable employee for 10 years and is not being supported by the leaders of that organization.

When a staff member has broken a policy, the administrator must seek to understand the context of the situation and validate the internal agreement that is present with the fellow employee. For instance, if a staff member refused to stay and care for a patient when there was a critical staffing need, before suspending the employee, a rule that exists in many organizations, it is crucial to understand why the employee refused to stay and why the staffing levels would not accommodate the need. If care providers have a by-the-book role model, then they see the value in following policies without regard to the context. Patients will eventually be at the receiving end of the same treatment.

Policies based on the symphonological approach would be written to allow leadership discretion for when to administer the written discipline, when to suspend an employee, etc. It is not possible to create the best practice environment on paper and still have a practice environment that works for patients and the clinical staff. It is essential that the leaders have developed to the point where they make appropriate decisions because they cannot fall back on the rules. This type of decision making is extremely important because the end result is an employee who feels she is treated with respect, who will then treat patients with the same respect because it is the nature of the environment. It also serves to produce the employee loyalty that is needed for well-coordinated organizational actions. Lack of congruence among the administrators regarding such issues leads to confusion and the search for more policies.

Summary

Symphonology can be used in administrative practice as a conceptual framework and decision-making process in much the same way that it is used in direct-care provision. Administrators have the same opportunity to make ethical decisions as direct-care providers and must be guided by the same framework if consistency is to exist in the organization.

II.   MANAGED CARE AND ETHICAL DECISION MAKING

The Current Managed Care Environment

In the United States in 1980, there were 235 Health Maintenance Organizations (HMOs) with an enrollment of 9.1 million members, which increased to 572

HMOs with 33 million members in 1990, and to 651 HMOs with 64.8 million members in 1998 (U.S. Census Bureau, 1999). Not only has the degree of managed care market penetration changed, but also the types of patient populations sought after by managed care organizations (MCOs). Over the past 5 years, in particular, there has been a notably increased interest in the Medicare and Medicaid managed care markets. Some states, such as Pennsylvania, have mandated the transition of their Medicaid program to managed care by contracting with third-party payers on a regional basis. This has significant implications for vulnerable populations and health care organizations.

As the pervasiveness of managed care has increased, so have the ethical problems associated with it. A few examples include dilemmas related to access to care, denial of medically necessary care, limited or complicated grievance/appeal processes available to consumers or providers, and delays in payments to providers that jeopardizes their financial viability and existence in the community. In response to this, consumer advocacy groups, hospital associations, and health care professional associations have become very active in lobbying both at the federal and state level. Thus, the national Patient Bill of Rights debate in Washington, D.C., and, at the state level, laws such as Pennsylvania Act 68 and the Quality Health Care Accountability Protection Act have been enacted. Despite legislative attempts to protect individual patients and large vulnerable populations, front-line health care administrators, professionals, and consumers struggle to deal with the effects of managed care in everyday practice.

The Health Care Provider's Fiscal Fiduciary/Patient Care Quandary

Health care organizations and professionals exist to provide care to patients. Therefore, as a benefactor of the community, it is the responsibility of a health care organization and its health care professionals to be fiscally viable and provide the highest quality of care to its patients. This poses a difficult challenge for health care providers, particularly in the managed care environment.

At the patient level, the health care professional has an implicit agreement with the patient to be their agent in meeting the patient's health care needs. Likewise, the patient agrees to be the patient (fulfilling his responsibilities in the treatment plan) and not placing unreasonable or unnecessary demands on the health care professional, particularly those outside the realm of the health care professional's scope of practice or control (i.e., the patient's social/economic situation). At times, the patient and health care professional may also have explicit agreements on how the patient's health care needs are to be met. Once these agreements have been made, the health care professional has a responsibility to fulfill the agreements unless the context of the patient's situation changes or the nature of the agreements change. Fulfilling these agreements, at times, will put health care professionals at odds with MCOs and/or the health care organization in which they work. As discussed below, symphonology can assist professionals in dealing with these dilemmas when they occur.

Payer Expectations and Challenges

Like health care provider organizations, health care payers and MCOs also have a fiscal fiduciary responsibility. Their responsibility is to their stockholders in the for-profit world or, in some not-for-profit cases, their Board of Trustees and the community at large. Briefly, MCOs expect *contracted* health care providers to provide the highest quality of *medically necessary* care for those members who are *eligible* for the specific service/benefit being provided. This sounds fairly straightforward, but it is far from it in reality.

For example, MCOs require all of their rules and requirements to be fulfilled by both the member (patient) and contracted provider for payment to occur. In other words, even if care is medically necessary, if a member or a provider makes a mistake in the procedure for authorizing the services rendered, MCOs can and do deny payment for that care. There are also times when an MCO makes mistakes in stating a patient's eligibility and authorizes patient admissions only to later say a mistake was made, when the patient really was not eligible for benefits and a denial of payment is made. Additionally, the most complicated and frustrating issue is that there are varying interpretations of what medically necessary care means from the respective patient, health care professional, and MCO perspectives. This can result in delays in or nonapproval of elective procedures/admissions. It also can lead to intense appeal processes for denials in reimbursement for care already rendered, such as emergency room care or the final days of an approved acute-care admission.

It is by no means the authors' intention to paint a picture that all MCOs behave unethically in all patient situations, as this is simply not true. There are many benefits to patients belonging to an HMO. In most situations, MCOs and health care professionals work collaboratively to effectively meet the needs of patients in an amicable manner. Unfortunately, at times, there are HMOs or personnel within HMOs that make poor decisions or have questionable practices. These questionable practices can put individual patient's health at risk or jeopardize health care organizations' financial viability. Conversely, there are times when the HMO and the health care professional concur on the patient's situation and the appropriate course of action. However, the patient and/or the patient's family do not agree with the course of action. This occurs, in most cases, due to the lack of objectivity or unrealistic expectations on their part and, therefore, they make out-of-context demands. In these situations, health care personnel are at odds with the patient rather than the MCO. It is in these types of individual cases that symphonology can assist the professional in everyday practice.

Application of Symphonology in the Managed Care Arena

First and foremost, the professional must understand and operate within the agreement. The implicit and explicit agreements between health care professionals and patients may vary depending on the context of the patient's situation, the type of professional involved in the situation, and the health care setting in which care is provided. For example, an intensive care nurse or case manager working in an acute-care hospital should not venture into the same types of agreements with a patient as a rehabilitation nurse or case manager working in a rehabilitation facility. Also, it would be unreasonable for a patient to expect or demand such agreements that are out of the health care professional's scope of practice or control. To illustrate this, it would be inappropriate for a physician or intensive care nurse to agree with a brain-injured patient (or the patient's family) that he would stay in the intensive care unit (ICU) setting until he is fully recovered. Agreeing to this would be clinically inappropriate for the patient. He would likely not receive the appropriate level of rehabilitation required for his recovery in an ICU setting. It would also be an unreasonably high cost for the organization to deliver a rehabilitation level of care in a costly ICU setting. This unnecessary cost would far exceed any reimbursement the health care organization would legitimately ever hope to get.

Second, the professional can benefit by understanding the ethical standards of autonomy, freedom, objectivity, self-assertion, beneficence, and fidelity, and utilizing them as lenses when evaluating a patient's situation, entering into agreements with patients, and making subsequent ethical decisions based on the health care professional patient agreements. In the brain-injured patient case above, if the patient/family are unable to objectively see the reality of the patient's situation, the health care professional has no obligation to enter into an agreement. Likewise, the professional may have no obligation to uphold an agreement in which the context of a situation has changed or there has been a loss of patient/ family objectivity subsequent to the agreement.

On the other hand, if a brain-injured patient who has rehabilitation potential is denied access to his rehabilitation benefits by an MCO, it is the professional's responsibility to fight/appeal the denial to the fullest extent on the patient's behalf to obtain the medically necessary services. This is typically a labor-intensive and time-consuming venture, but it is the only ethical decision to make. The involved professional cannot take the attitude of: "Oh well, we cannot do that procedure because the HMO will not pay for it." This decision is based primarily on the bioethical standards of the professional's autonomy, beneficence, and self-assertion. If the patient were able to act on his own behalf, he would expend his time and energy (self-assertion) to obtain the benefit of rehabilitation services so that he could return to his highest level of agency. Since he is unable to act on his own behalf, based on the professional/patient agreement, the professional is obligated to act for him.

The professional is bombarded in practice on a daily basis with conflicting responsibilities and demands on her time. This alone can be a great challenge and place the professional in an ethical dilemma. An additional way symphonology can assist the professional in daily practice is in triaging risks and benefits in each individual patient's situation and helping her prioritize how she spends her time with individual patients. Likewise, it can assist her in seeking out solutions, particularly in managed care cases, which mutually benefit both the patient and the health care organization. Financial viability of the organization is beneficial to the community and future patients who will be dependent on the organization to meet their health care needs through clinical programs and services.

Case Example

Mrs. Jones is a multiple trauma patient who is 26 weeks gestational and, while not brain dead, is in a persistent, unresponsive state. Following several weeks of acute care, Mrs. Jones' HMO determines she no longer requires acute care and should be transferred to a skilled nursing facility. Therefore, the HMO's per diem reimbursement will end immediately.

In addition to providing acute care to the patient, the health care team was also providing acute care to maintain viability of the unborn child until a time of safe delivery, which is what the patient's wishes would be according to the patient's husband/family. It is the medical team's assessment that the necessary monitoring and care to maintain the unborn child could not be provided in a skilled nursing facility. Thus, transferring Mrs. Jones would endanger the well being of the fetus. Mrs. Jones' Nurse Case Manager sought advice from her administrative director on how to resolve this ethical dilemma.

Following a discussion on the health care professional/patient agreement and the ethical standards, it is agreed, based on information from Mrs. Jones' family, that Mrs. Jones, if she were able to act on her own behalf, would do all she could to maintain the life of her unborn child. Therefore, the case manager is ethically responsible through the health care professional/patient agreement to do for Mrs. Jones that which she cannot do for herself. A solution is needed that benefits the patient, the unborn child, and, hopefully, the organization as well, or at least will minimize the risk to the organization.

Despite not knowing the ultimate financial impact of the decision, Mrs. Jones is kept in the acute care facility, where care for her and her unborn child are continued at the medically necessary level. In the interim, the case manager should appeal the HMO's decision to discontinue payment for acute care. The case manager should obtain all of the necessary documentation with the help of the medical team to demonstrate the medical necessity of acute care in order to win the appeal and avoid a negative financial impact on the hospital. If unsuccessful with the appeal process, the case manager should then negotiate a skilled reimbursement rate with the payer in order to keep Mrs. Jones at the acute care facility while at least minimizing the negative financial impact on the organization.

Summary

The daily challenges in the managed care environment can be extremely frustrating and stressful. There are days when the health care professional feels as if all she does is fight with MCOs for what is rightfully due to, and medically necessary for, individual patients. There are other times when patients and/or their families are not objective, and make unrealistic or unreasonable demands on the health care professional or do not maintain fidelity to the professional/patient agreement. As demonstrated above, symphonology can assist the professional in navigating these turbulent waters. By applying symphonology in everyday practice, the professional will have the greatest certainty that she is making ethically sound decisions that benefit her patients, as well as the organization in which she works. Organizations that empower and support ethical decision making among their health care professionals will benefit in the long term, as their reputation in the community for excellent practice will enable them to prosper.

REFERENCES

Benner, P., Tanner, C. A., & Chesla, C. A. (1996). *Expertise in nursing practice, caring, clinical judgment, and ethics.* New York: Springer.

Borawski, D. B. (1995). Ethical dilemmas for nurse administrators. *Journal of Nursing Administration, 25*(7/8), 60–62.

Camunas, C. (1994a). Ethical dilemmas of nurse executives, Part 1. *Journal of Nursing Administration, 24*(7/8), 45–51.

Camunas, C. (1994b). Ethical dilemmas of nurse executives continued, Part 2. *Journal of Nursing Administration, 25*(9), 19–23.

Chown, E. (1992). Managerial ethics. In S. A. Ziebarth (Ed.), *Feeling the squeeze: The practice of middle management in Canadian health care facilities* (pp. 37–45). Ottawa, Canada: Canadian Hospital Association.

Sietsema, M. R., & Spradley, B. W. (1987). Ethics and administrative decision making. *Journal of Nursing Administration, 17*(4), 28–32.

U.S. Census Bureau. (1999). *Statistical abstract of the United States: 1999* (119th ed.). Washington, DC: Author.

Wilson, D. M. (1998). Administrative decision making in response to sudden health care agency funding reductions: Is there a role for ethics? *Nursing Ethics, 5*, 319–329.

CHAPTER *14*

The Researcher/Subject Agreement

Barbara A. Brown

The use of symphonology as a research ethic begins, of course, with the agreement between the researcher and subject. However, in the case of a research study, the agreement is more than implicit. It is, and must be, made explicit. This is done through informed consent. Where the health care professional/patient agreement is sufficient to make attention to the bioethical standards necessary, in the researcher/subject agreement, the necessity of informed consent brings the standards to a more explicit level. Informed consent includes all of the bioethical standards in the researcher/subject relationship.

The Researcher/Subject Agreement and the Bioethical Standards

The relationship of the bioethical standards to this relationship would appear as follows:

Fidelity in the research relationship is faithfulness to the agreement that is explicated in the gaining of informed consent. For this relationship, it is best to begin with fidelity and work toward autonomy, rather than vice versa.

Beneficence in research is based on a harm/benefit analysis. Few would voluntarily enter into an agreement in which the harms would outweigh the benefits. The most important risks and benefits are those that affect the participant and must be explicated in the process of gaining consent. Although the harm/benefit ratio must be outlined by the researcher, a subject can ultimately decide if he is willing to risk possible harms for a specific benefit. This benefit is not always realized by the subject. This must be made clear so that the subject can make an informed choice. Finally, the researcher is obligated to stop the experiment at any stage if there is reason to believe that the participant may experience unforseen harm or even death if the experiment continues.

Self-assertion is upheld by allowing the participant, at every stage in the research, to control, to whatever extent is possible, his own time and effort. This begins with the forming of the agreement, an agreement that "is attained by voluntary consent, objectively gained." Valid consent is free of coercion and undue influence. If the nature of the study requires limitations placed on the participant's time and effort, then these must be made very clear in the informed-consent process. The idea of self-assertion should also be taken into account in the manner in which the researcher chooses research participants. Those who have lost control of much of their own time and effort (i.e., those who are institutionalized) should not be the only groups to bear the burden of research. Unfortunately, in the past, these groups were used in large numbers because of the convenience of obtaining the sample, and sufficient consideration was not given to their rights.

Objectivity, in this case, must be "the whole truth and nothing but the truth." Information cannot be withheld for any reason. The subject must have complete and truthful information upon which to decide whether to participate in the study. That is, given the necessary information to make an informed decision in a manner that adapts the information given to the capacities of the participant.

Freedom is maintained by giving the subject the right to make voluntary choices, to choose to participate or not participate in the study, and also to choose to continue or not once the study has begun. This must be done in such a way that there is no coercion whatsoever. The subject must understand that care will not change regardless of whether he participates in the study.

Autonomy functions somewhat differently in this relationship. The research subject is usually chosen because of his similarity to other subjects. This similarity has a direct connection to the purpose of the research study itself. A person's specific uniqueness as an individual is not the focus. However, this does not mean that the researcher should be unaware of the individual subject. For example, there are times when, because of the particular uniqueness of a person, the researcher should not consider a particular person as a potential research subject.

Discussion

Research for participants who cannot give their own consent (such as children, the mentally retarded, the mentally ill, those suffering from dementia, etc.) must be undertaken with extreme caution. It is essential, however, to do research on these groups in the hope of gaining information to improve their conditions or of those who have the same condition. Thus, the consent of surrogates is accepted where there is minimal chance of harm. With children especially, the research must have, at least, some potential to directly benefit them (Lo, 2000). It is important to remember that people who cannot give their own consent have not told us what they are willing to risk and what they are willing to endure. "Vulnerable, disadvantaged, or minority groups should be neither over-represented in dangerous studies nor under-represented in trials of promising new therapies" (Lo, 2000, p. 222).

The researcher has the responsibility to design a worthwhile study, to see that all of the requirements of Institutional Review Boards are met, and to exert caution in recruiting and using subjects. During the study itself, the researcher has an obligation to monitor what is happening, and to be aware of what is going on with the people involved, so that at any given moment a person could be withdrawn from the study as the evidence warrants. In the publishing of the study, the researcher must be true to the data, be sensitive to confidentiality issues, identify appropriate authors, and acknowledge funding sources, if any.

REFERENCE

Lo, B. (2000). *Resolving ethical dilemmas: A guide for clinicians* (2nd ed.). Philadelphia: Lippincott, Williams, & Wilkins.

CHAPTER 15

The Professional/Patient Agreement and Advance Directives

Barbara A. Brown

The Patient Self-Determination Act (PSDA) was a federally mandated step to acknowledge patient rights to either refuse or accept treatment (Omnibus Budget Reconciliation Act, 1990). Primarily, the PSDA mandated that patients (or potential patients as in the case of managed care services) receive information concerning end-of-life decisions, their right to refuse medical care, and, subsequently, their right to formulate advance directives. It was thought that the PSDA would not only increase the ethical power of self-determination of consumers (an ethical right of every person to control his own destiny) through advance directives, but also provide a mechanism for controlling health care costs and for correcting the balance between health care consumers and providers. Unfortunately, these outcomes have not been realized (Reich, 1995). Among the reasons given for this lack of success are that people do not want to discuss end-of-life issues, some fear that they will not receive the same quality of care, the language is difficult to comprehend, and there is little or no education done to help people draft an advance directive (Rein et al., 1996).

Education and discussion concerning advance directives (living wills and durable power of attorneys for care) are essential in the process of the execution of these documents (Hoffman & Gill, 2000; Waters, 2000).

GUIDANCE THROUGH THE BIOETHICAL STANDARDS

Advance directives assist the health care professional in establishing an objective awareness of the patient and understanding the difference, from the patient's point of view, between what is beneficial and what is harmful. The agreement made in any advance directive, whether it be a living will or a durable power of attorney for health care, is one that has as its foundation the bioethical standards. The bioethical standards serve as a lens through which the person's desires can be viewed. They form the ethical basis that are embodied in an advance directive, therefore, they help show people what an advance directive can provide for them when they no longer can speak for themselves and give guidance to professionals in carrying out the wishes of their patients.

Autonomy—Autonomy has the most bearing on advance directives. It maintains a keystone position in relation to the other bioethical standards. Advance directives are a means by which persons maintain their autonomy, their sense of self, even if they become incompetent.

Freedom—In the health care setting, freedom is obtained in three ways: informed consent, substituted judgment standard (that considers the person's own desires), or best interest standard that considers the person's sameness or humanness and is used when it is not known what the person desires. In all cases, informed consent is the preferred method, but is not possible for an incompetent person. Substituted judgment is the next, most preferred method, and one that an advance directive makes possible by obtaining information regarding the patient's wishes while the person can still reason about them.

Objectivity—Advance directives provide a way for the patient to communicate his objective evaluation of the facts to the health care professional. However, the context changes, so what the patient expresses can only be tentative. This is why it is sometimes necessary for the health care professional to interpret the advance directive in order to act objectively and contextually—providing the care for the incompetent patient that the patient would want if he could reflect on the situation with full knowledge. This is very difficult to do at times. This is where a durable power of attorney for health care (proxy) can help interpret what the patient would want.

Self-assertiveness—Advance directives protect the right of a patient to control his time and effort (e.g., prevent futile care that a person does not want).

Beneficence—The person, in his advance directive, can make known his ideas regarding what is beneficial and harmful from his own unique perspective.

Fidelity—The patient expects that a health care professional will be faithful to his wishes as stated in his advance directive. To adhere to the terms of the advance directive, albeit contextually, means to adhere to the terms of an agreement. This sometimes means to the spirit, rather than the letter, of the advance directive.

THE PROBLEM OF INTERPRETATION

When a person has drafted an advance directive with little or no education and discussion before checking off what they want and do not want, or has not appointed a proxy (or the proxy is no longer capable of making those decisions), the problem of interpretation becomes, in many cases, difficult (Campbell, 1995). Just what would this person want in this circumstance? Because education about the drafting of advance directives is sparse or nonexistent, people often are not well-informed about their choices and the consequences of their choices, frequently they do not even know what they have stipulated (Danis, Garrett, Harris, & Patrick, 1994; Fischer, Alpert, Stoeckle, & Emanuel, 1997). While there are times when a person's advance directive is not being followed and it should be, there are other times when, in the context of the situation, it is hard to see how this person would want the health care professional to follow the letter of his advance directive. Patients trust professionals to follow the spirit of their intentions (New Jersey State Nurses' Association, 1999). For instance, a person gets stung by a bee and goes into respiratory arrest, but he has an advance directive that says he is not to be intubated. What would the spirit of his advance directive permit the health care professional to do?

CONTEXT

Advance directives act as contextual guidelines. They bring to the situation the patient's context of knowledge (e.g., his beliefs and attitudes). This must be considered in order to relate the decision to the patient's desires, purposes, and actions. Advance directives become the fiber that is woven into the formation of the context. They are a significant part of the context when a person is unable to speak for himself regarding treatment decisions. Advance directives enable health care professionals to understand the context of the patient in the context of the situation. But the limitation of an advance directive, as stated before, is that the person cannot evaluate the present situation in light of his values and beliefs. Patients trust us to do for them what they would do for themselves. We must, and this must be done with caution and thought, act in accordance with the spirit of what they have said they want and interpret their words in light of the context. This is fidelity to the agreement.

CONCLUSION

The bioethical standards serve as a framework that supports advance directives. Advanced directives emanate from the agreement between the patient and the health care professional. Their very existence depends upon the interweaving of the context of the situation and the context of knowledge of the participants. Symphonology can be used to create a discussion guide to help educate people about the value of advance directives and then allow them to make an educated choice about what they wish to do.

The following is offered as a discussion guide that health care professionals can use with patients (Brown, 1998). (The reader must bear in mind that the specific questions and how the questions are asked depends on the person and the situation. Therefore, the reader must make the necessary adjustments.)

One could begin the discussion in this way: An advance directive is an agreement between you and your health care providers that they will give you the care you desire. It is a way for you to maintain your unique desires and decide on what you do and do not want done when you can no longer tell us. An advance directive protects you from receiving treatments that you would refuse if you were able or from not receiving treatments you would want if you could state your wishes. Talk to me about what is important to you—what are your thoughts? Here the medical directive is useful because it gives various scenarios, and the person can choose: given this, I want that, given that, I want this (Emanuel & Emanuel, 1989). It requires a health care professional to go over the form with the person. It is time consuming, but it is worth the time. Regardless of what form is used, it is necessary that the health care professional discuss it with the patient and interpret the choices in light of the person's desires and present circumstances.

What kinds of things would you consider beneficial? (Follow-up questions are necessary and depend on the person's responses). Under what circumstances would you want treatment continued or discontinued? Would you like to appoint a proxy (durable power of attorney for health care) to help us make decisions for you? This person can look at what is happening and reflect your choices—given the situation at the time.

A discussion of this type, of course, is incomplete, because the situation must guide the discussion. However, it shows how symphonology can and does direct discussions with patients, and not just in the area of advance directives.

REFERENCES

Brown, B. (1998). Factors influencing the drafting of advance directives by elders: A quasi-experiment study. Unpublished Doctoral Dissertation, Duquesne University, Pittsburgh, PA.

Campbell, M. (1995). Interpretation of an ambiguous advance directive. *Dimensions of Critical Care Nursing, 14*, 226–232.

Danis, M., Garrett, J., Harris, R., & Patrick, D. (1994). Stability of choices about life-sustaining treatments. *Annals of Internal Medicine, 120*, 567–573.

Emanuel, L., & Emanuel, E. (1989). The medical directive. *Journal of the AMA, 261,* 3288–3293.

Fischer, G. S., Alpert, H. R., Stoeckle, J. D., & Emanuel, L. L. (1997). Can goals of care be used to predict intervention preferences in an advance directive? *Archives of Internal Medicine, 157,* 801–807.

Hoffman, I. J., & Gill, B. (2000). Beginning with the end in mind. *American Journal of Nursing, 00*(5) (Suppl.), 38–41, 47–50.

New Jersey State Nurses' Association. (1999). NJSNA position statement: The nurses's role in the end of life decision making. *New Jersey Nurse, 29*(8), 10.

Omnibus Budget Reconciliation Act. (1990). PL 101-508 *Congressional Record,* October 26, 1990.

Reich, W. (Ed.). (1995). *Advance directives: Encyclopedia of bioethics* (Rev. ed.). New York: Macmillan.

Rein, A., Harshman, D., Frick, T., Phillips, J., Lewis, S., & Nolan, M. (1996). Advance directive decision making among medical inpatients. *Journal of Professional Nursing, 12*(1), 39–46.

Waters, C. M. (2000). End of life care directives among African Americans: Lessons learned—a need for community-centered discussion and education. *Journal of Community Health Nursing, 17*(1), 25–37.

Case Study Analyses

Analyses of Dilemmas

A NOTE TO THE READER

In going over these dilemmas, the reader should recall that they are abstract case studies. In abstract case studies, of course, it sounds as though the nature of the case is very clear and the responsibility of any health care professional is equally clear and rigid. In the context of a real-life situation, however, a health care professional seldom enjoys this clarity.

It is possible that, for one or more dilemmas, a reader may come to a different resolution than the resolution given here. This is not surprising. There is no real-world context to which to refer. Everyone approaches a dilemma from the perspective of recent experiences, ideas, and attitudes. A nurse may unconsciously rewrite the dilemma from her perspective. Or it is possible to add something to the context that is not given in the dilemma. **A different perspective or context may, very logically, result in a different resolution to this new and different dilemma.** The reader is asked to perform a thought experiment: Without changing anything of the dilemma as it is given, form a different perspective to the dilemma in your mind—one that suggests the resolution given. This will significantly sharpen your understanding of ethical decision making.

A simple example of this:

> John is in the hospital. The hospital is notified that John's wife has died. John's nurse, Emma, is elected to tell him of his wife's death.

One possible resolution: Emma should tell John at this time.
Another possible resolution: Emma should not tell John at this time.

If one assumes that John would suffer no harm by being told at this time, or might be benefitted in some objective way, one would come to the first resolution.

If one assumes that John might suffer harm by being told at this time, and would not be benefitted, one would come to the second resolution.

Not all dilemmas will be this simple. But many will be. Even in this dilemma, background information is necessary to its justifiable resolution.

There is a very large difference between a real-life context and a case study. Nothing that follows should instill a feeling of ethical incompetence in the reader. Many of the following dilemmas are highly context dependent. In addition, some are quite difficult. Several are dilemmas nurses or other health care personnel meet in their interactions with physicians. These usually are more difficult to resolve than dilemmas that only involve patients.

While most of the dilemmas only involve nurses, not all of them do. Some involve other professionals, such as physicians, pharmacists, physical therapists, social workers, dieticians, psychologists, etc.

The final resolutions of some of these dilemmas can be discovered only in the actual context in which they arise. All that can be done in a case study analysis is to make the nature of the dilemmas clear. In some cases, we will offer only broad suggestions as to the direction the resolutions might take.

The purpose of these analyses is to make the reader stronger and more knowledgeable. Many ethical agents do not allow themselves to know when their response to an ethical situation has been inadequate. Without knowledge, there is no growth. Without growth, there is no possibility of consistently appropriate ethical decision making. It is a nurse's responsibility to know. The purpose of these resolutions is to enable the reader to orient her or his thinking about bioethical matters and to develop, over time, competence and confidence at ethical decision making.

ANALYSES

Dilemma 1-1, page 13   What to do when a patient's right to know conflicts with his desire not to know.

It is a rule that a patient has a right to know the details of his condition. When Zelda relates all this to Mr. Wu, she obeys the rule and satisfies Mr. Wu. There are times when a patient must be told the details of his condition. This is necessary in order that he can understand and make decisions concerning his course of treatment. If Zelda had informed Mr. Wu, not on the basis of a rule but on the basis of analysis, and the realization that this action on her part was appropriate, there is no way in which Mr. Wu could have been worse off. The fact that she did it on the basis of its being a rule in no way increased its benefit to Mr. Wu.

It is quite conceivable that had she taken the action on the basis of analysis, she might have done it more effectively, she might have guided her actions more skillfully. But a practitioner of duty has no reason to be concerned with the skills that might be developed through analysis.

Let us see if we can find a bioethical standard to justify Zelda's relating this information to Mr. Goldfarb:

Autonomy: Mr. Goldfarb's nature is such that he does not desire this detailed information. Having this information does not do him any good. At the same time, it does him some harm.

If a patient's primary reason for entering the health care system is to receive information, then perhaps Mr. Goldfarb's autonomy would have a lessened relevance. In entering the health care system, it might be said, that he consents to receive the information. If a patient's primary reason for entering the health care system was to receive information, the majority of patients who come into the hospital would discover the details of their condition and leave. Such is not the case. The primary reason for a patient's entering the health care system is to regain his physical or psychological well-being. Zelda violated Mr. Goldfarb's autonomy.

Freedom: Mr. Goldfarb has a right to know. A patient has the right to know because knowing enables him to take informed action. If knowing does not enable him to take informed action, then knowing has little value. Knowing has no value for Mr. Goldfarb. His right to take action is prior to, and logically more important than, his right to know. His purpose (health and well-being) is more important than information for its own sake.

In addition to his right to know, Mr. Goldfarb has a right not to know. This right ought to especially be respected when his not knowing **assists** his freedom of action and his well-being better than his being informed. Zelda's exercise of complete freedom takes away all of Mr. Goldfarb's freedom. There are others, not so morally fastidious, who could tell Mr. Goldfarb what he needs to know. Zelda is taking the place of a nurturing nurse.

Objectivity: Every truth that a nurse relates to a patient should be treated like a wild horse. It should always be controlled by beneficence.

The detailed truths that Zelda related to Mr. Goldfarb were not motivated by maleficence. However, Zelda should have been guided by beneficence and she was not. The standard of objectivity offers her no justification.

Approaching the question of objectivity through Zelda's eyes utterly undermines objectivity. In the health care system, objectivity is not simply having information, but being able to act effectively on the information one has. It is much better that Mr. Goldfarb's course of action be guided by objectivity rather than have it undermined by information.

Self-assertion: In order that people, in their interactions, do not aggress against each other, there must be an agreement between them to respect each other's self-ownership. Ethically, no one can be involved in an interaction unless he has given his consent. One person cannot influence the action of another person without the consent of that other person unless he takes over the ownership of that other person.

Try to imagine someone controlling the action of a pair of scissors without controlling the pair of scissors.

Between Zelda and Mr. Goldfarb, as between every nurse and patient, there is an implicit agreement that each will respect the self-ownership of the other. Zelda violated that agreement. In his condition, Mr. Goldfarb needs the power to exercise self-assertion.

Beneficence: Zelda did Mr. Goldfarb harm for the sake of doing that which did no good. Perhaps Zelda did not know the effect that her action would have on Mr. Goldfarb. If she did not know, she should have known. She cannot appeal to the standard of beneficence.

Fidelity: Zelda was faithful to the standard of fidelity just in case the nurse/patient agreement involves a nurse's taking particular actions regardless of their consequences. The nurse/patient agreement, of course, does not involve this. Zelda can find no support in the standard of fidelity.

Dilemma 1-2, page 16   Should a dying patient's desire for confidentiality override his family's plans for a pleasant surprise?

The bioethical standards are principles of the nurse/patient agreement. The standard of self-assertion requires Harry's nurse to reveal the fact of his son's return and let Harry decide what he desires to do. Nonetheless, we will analyze the dilemma in terms of the other bioethical standards.

Autonomy: Harry's nurse must keep her agreement with her patient. If she could know that Harry's character-structure was such that he would prefer his family's knowing in order that he might enjoy the surprise, then perhaps she should inform his family. This would not be for utilitarian reasons, but for Harry's benefit and in keeping with their agreement. At all odds, it is very unlikely that Harry's nurse could have any certain knowledge of this. Therefore, it almost certainly should not determine her decision.

Freedom: Harry's life story will be enhanced through his knowing that his son is coming home.

Objectivity: If Harry believes that his nurse will not advise his family of his prognosis, and she does, then she violates the standard of objectivity by undermining Harry's objective awareness.

In the nature of the case, she cannot ask for Harry's advice. She cannot ask him whether he wants to know that his son is coming home without letting him know that his son is coming home.

Self-assertion: Harry will have better control of how he wants to use his time and effort.

Beneficence: There is no sense in which the standard of beneficence calls for a nurse to do the greatest good for the greatest number. It calls for her to do the greatest good for her patient. Harry's nurse does this by going to Harry and discussing the situation with him.

Fidelity: The nurse can assume that Harry would desire to know that his son is safe and coming home. This knowledge would enhance the remainder of his life and, perhaps, even make the dying process easier for Harry. This is the nurse's professional responsibility.

A nurse's one overriding agreement is with her patient. Fidelity requires that she be true to this agreement. The nurse/patient agreement will not allow Harry's nurse to do nothing. She must discuss the situation either with Harry or with his family. She cannot discuss it with his family without Harry's permission. She must discuss it with Harry.

She might begin somewhat like this: "Harry, I want you to let me tell your family about your condition. There are a number of things they will want to discuss with you. Harry, I am going to ask you to trust me. Honest to God, if you let me talk to them, you will be very glad you did." However, Harry **must** know of his son's homecoming.

Dilemma 2-1, page 21   Should a nurse feed a stroke patient who must learn to feed himself?

This dilemma calls for Yvonne to ascertain ethical balance and proportion. If the long-term physical and emotional effects of feeding himself exceed the short-term effects of his not feeding himself, then Steve should feed himself. If the short-term effects outweigh the long-term effects, then Yvonne should feed him.

Yvonne should refer to the context of the dilemma. There will be a short-term demoralizing effect on Steve if he feeds himself. There will be a long-term enhancement of his life and purposes in beginning to feed himself now.

Yvonne must, in order to discover the best decision, weigh and measure one against the other, and act on the basis of balance and proportion.

Dilemma 2-2, page 21   Are there circumstances under which a nurse is justified in discontinuing home visits?

Looking at it as a type of triage situation (triage, as a method of ethical analysis, is discussed in chapter 3 on page 56), we have this: If Martin's time and effort could be better given to other patients, and because Frank has broken the nurse/patient agreement with Martin, Martin is justified in discussing discontinuing home visits with Frank's physician.

Dilemma 2-3, page 22   What is the relative importance of protocol versus patients?

Nearly always when a context is distorted and misread, it is because it has been "widened" beyond its relevant contours. The situation can also appear problematic if the context is narrowed too stringently. On the one hand, the patient needs attention that she cannot be given in Josh's location. On the other hand, hospital policy and practice requires that an attending physician sign a transfer order. Looking at it from the narrow perspective, then, is no way to resolve it.

But the context of the situation is formed by purposes that are to be accomplished in the health care setting. And that is not possible here. A wider context must be sought. It must be sought in the context of knowledge.

The primary elements of the context of knowledge is formed by the nature and definition of the roles of those engaged in seeking to achieve the purpose. In this case, it is the definition of a physician, a nurse, and a patient.

However a physician is defined, the purposes of the physician that do not involve the welfare of patients are far less important than the purposes that do. These latter are the **defining** purposes of the physician and the entire health care system.

The only ethical course for Josh to follow is to transfer Mrs. Allison to the other hospital. And then depend on the calm, modest, rational objectivity of the physician. This attitude of the physician is the only ethical attitude possible to her. **The ethical responsibilities of any professional are set out in the definition of her profession.**

Dilemma 2-4, page 35   Should a physician order beneficial surgery against a patient's wishes?

Autonomy: Harold is unique. His motivations for refusing the amputation of his gangrenous leg must certainly be unique. But they are his motivations; it is his leg and his life. The physician, apparently, did not ask Harold why he was refusing the operation. Or, if she did, Harold's answer did not satisfy her.

Harold's motivations and values are unique. So are the motivations and values of the physician. In order for Harold's answer to satisfy the physician, their motivations and values would have to be harmonious. If Harold's answer must satisfy his physician, then Harold's physician has the same rights in relation to Harold's life as Harold has. In fact, this would give the physician not only the same rights, but greater rights than Harold.

As one human to another, the physician has a right, as a health care professional, to exert gentle coercion. But since Harold is an autonomous individual, by right, he has no ethical responsibility to satisfy his physician on a decision concerning an operation that he does not want.

Freedom: The physician's action is an attack on Harold's freedom of choice in the matter of his own life. If this freedom is taken away, Harold has no freedom left. Without freedom, there is no possibility of Harold acting ethically. There is no possibility of Harold acting at all. Because Harold cannot engage in ethical actions, he cannot engage in ethical interactions. And, therefore, Harold's physician cannot be engaged in an ethical interaction with Harold.

The ethical choice that the physician is forcing on Harold is not a choice. Harold cannot choose because Harold cannot think and decide for himself. It is not possible for any person to think, decide, or choose when a course of action is forced upon him.

Harold's physician believes that her course of action is best for Harold, despite Harold's disagreement. The course of her ethical development was arrested too soon. A higher level of ethical development would produce the belief that no interaction can be justified unless that interaction is chosen by free ethical agents with an equal ethical status, and, in her case, on the basis of a professional agreement.

Objectivity: This dilemma does not involve the standard of objectivity:

1. It does not involve Harold's physician attempting to deceive him.
2. Harold has no ethical responsibility, in this context, to tell his physician any truth. Harold's physician has no right to expect Harold to tell her any truth that would assist the physician in her aggression against Harold's rights.

Self-assertion: A health care professional does not protect a patient's right to self-assertion by destroying it.

Beneficence: To destroy a patient's individual sovereignty is not to act beneficently toward him. There is no such thing as acting beneficently toward a person by giving him a benefit he does not want.

H. G. Wells wrote a story called "The Richest Man in Bogota." This is the story of a man whose airplane crashes in a valley among the mountains of Columbia. In the crash, the man loses the sight of one of his eyes. The valley where he crashes is filled with diamonds. The brilliance of these diamonds has made everyone who lives in the valley blind. When the inhabitants of the valley discover what has happened to the airplane pilot, they decide that they must put out his other eye. They are all very happy not being sighted. They do not suffer the glare of the diamonds. They believe that anyone who can look out upon the valley must suffer from the glare. So they decide they will blind the pilot, out of beneficence, for his own benefit.

Coercive beneficence cannot be beneficence.

Fidelity: Ask yourself if you would enter into an agreement with a physician if one of the terms of that agreement allowed the physician unlimited freedom to do anything she wanted.

Analysis through the bioethical standards does not justify the physician's actions.

Dilemma 3-1, page 44   What should be done with a patient who refuses an appendectomy?

The first thing Anthony should do is try to discover Mr. Nathan's reason for refusing the operation. If Mr. Nathan has a reason, this must be dealt with and, quite possibly, accepted. On the face of it, however, it is difficult to imagine what that reason might be.

Autonomy: It may be that Mr. Nathan's desire not to have the operation expresses his autonomy. But autonomy, being the expression of a person's individual nature, usually would not take this form. It is not evident how Mr. Nathan's desire serves the best interest of his rational nature or of his animal nature. It may be that Mr. Nathan is out of touch with his human nature and unable to express his autonomy.

Freedom: Mr. Nathan has a right to take a free, uncoerced action. Although his action, to be an action, must be an expression of whom Mr. Nathan is in his present life context. If Anthony exerts gentle coercion, this might, so to speak, bring Mr. Nathan to himself and make it possible for him to exercise a capacity for free action, which he has lost.

Objectivity: There is not one truth for Mr. Nathan and another truth for Anthony. In this situation, as in every situation, there is only one truth. This truth may not be easy to discover. And Mr. Nathan and Anthony might draw different conclusions concerning it. The truth may be such that it is reasonable for Mr. Nathan to refuse the operation. This would be so unusual that it would be a failure of responsibility on Anthony's part simply to assume it.

Anthony has the delicate task of discovering the truth, helping Mr. Nathan to discover it, and avoiding the temptation to justify a violation of Mr. Nathan's rights by a process of rationalization. Anthony's professional responsibility calls on him to guide himself—and Mr. Nathan—in the pursuit of the greatest benefit.

Self-assertion: Mr. Nathan has a right to control his time and effort. He has uttered a word of refusal concerning the operation. But this refusal is so unusual that it is reasonable to question whether it expresses Mr. Nathan's actual desire. Not to question Mr. Nathan's communication would be a failure of the nurse/patient agreement. Anthony's agreement is pledged to the well-being of Mr. Nathan. It is an agreement to act as Mr. Nathan's agent. Anthony cannot fulfill this agreement by being passive and perfectly acquiescent.

Authoritarianism would lead to ignoring Mr. Nathan's rights and desires and aggressively operating on him. An extreme form of "libertarianism" would, without hesitation, lead to accepting Mr. Nathan's refusal. This mindless, deontological form of fidelity would be unquestioning fidelity to a word—fidelity to a "No."

Beneficence: An unheeding beneficence to Mr. Nathan cannot be an aggression that ignores what he is communicating. But neither can it be an indifference that ignores his human nature and the nature of the human condition and does not question what he is communicating. Beneficence must be based on communicating with Mr. Nathan—and **with his context.**

Fidelity: A biomedical professional's fidelity is fidelity to a person—to a reasoning animal, but to a specific person in a specific situation.

Dilemma 3-2, page 54 **What should the health professional do when a patient delays life-saving treatment to protect the life of her unborn child?**

The fact that Mabel is lying to herself has great ethical relevance in this context.

Autonomy: By lying to herself, Mabel has closed off her autonomy to Charlene. In refusing to consider one or more relevant factors, Mabel takes herself out of any objective context. She has broken the connection between the context of knowledge and the context of her situation. She has broken the connection between Charlene and herself. Mabel presents no autonomy and no objective context with which Charlene can deal.

Mabel has not considered the fact that the two outcomes open to her are opposed to each other. She cannot have the child and fight her cancer. Mabel can establish an objective context only by considering all the alternative possibilities and choosing one.

The fact that she is unwilling to consider every possibility makes it difficult or impossible for Charlene to communicate with her.

Freedom: Mabel is unwilling to make an objective judgment based on every alternative open to her. Under these circumstances, she cannot engage in free action. She has bound herself. Charlene cannot try to influence her freedom. She has given up her freedom.

Objectivity: Charlene owes Mabel the truth. A patient also has some responsibility to give truthful communications to the health care professionals caring for her. Mabel is violating this standard. This gives Charlene no basis for effective ethical action.

Self-assertion: Mabel is using her self-assertion to protect herself against the reality of her situation. She is defending herself against the value of the counsel that Charlene could give her.

Beneficence: Mabel is walled off from the influence of Charlene and other health care professionals. Under the circumstances, beneficence is not possible.

In order for Charlene to benefit Mabel, Mabel will have to analyze her situation and apply some level of reason to the course of action she decides on. Mabel seems entirely unwilling or unable to do this.

Fidelity: In this narrow aspect of their relationship, there is no communication between Mabel and Charlene. Since there is no communication, there is no agreement other than the most basic nurse/patient agreement. In everything outside of this dilemma, Charlene owes Mabel fidelity. Mabel's method of resolving this dilemma, however, is so inappropriate that Charlene has nothing to give her fidelity to in this situation.

Charlene ought to help Mabel in everything she can. In the context of this dilemma, until Mabel becomes willing to open herself up to all the alternatives of her situation, there is little Charlene can do.

The bioethical standards have been of little help in resolving this dilemma. For the bioethical standards to be significantly helpful, a patient must be willing to consider all the relevant facts.

Dilemma 4-1, page 62   Should a patient in a persistent vegetative state be allowed to die?

All four arguments are misleading:

The unique individual that he once was does still exist. The state of being that he once enjoyed, however, no longer exists. Even if it were true to say that, "The autonomous individual no longer exists," nothing would follow from this. If anything ought to be done, this can only be because an autonomous individual does exist. If an autonomous individual does not exist, then there is nothing that must be done.

- There is no way that anyone can benefit this patient. What should be done cannot be determined by beneficence. There is no way to exercise beneficence in relation to this patient.
- Life is not precious to him. Nothing is or can be of any value to him. If a tribute can be paid to him and to his life, that tribute might be his death, as well as his continued existence.
- The notion of autonomy involves three notions—uniqueness, rational animality, and ethical equality.

As a rational animal, the patient is specifically identical to every other human individual. Therefore, he is ethically the equal of every other human individual. Autonomy also involves ethical equality.

It is true that no one has a right to terminate the life of an autonomous individual. This is not because an autonomous individual is unique. It is not because, when he is observed, he appears different from other people. An autonomous individual acquires the right to life through the fact that he is a rational animal.

Every person and the context of every person is unique. Certain general principles, such as the individual person's independence, must guide every action in any context similar to this. Consideration must also be given to the actual differences that exist in the context.

In this person's context, there are four relevant differences:

1. He has requested that he be allowed to die.
2. He is now permanently dependent on the efforts of others.
3. None of the elements of human autonomy now characterize him. He is conscious of no desires; he is totally out of touch with the world. He engages in no reasoning processes, nor will he ever. His life consists in basic physiological processes; this is not autonomous. He has no purposes. He has no power to exercise agency.
4. Allowing his life to terminate is not the same as terminating his life.

The recognition of this patient's autonomy does not speak against allowing him to die. The bioethical standards do not demand that he be kept alive.

Dilemma 4-2, page 66   **What should a pharmacist and nurse do when a resident refuses to change a prescription they believe may be harmful to the patient?**

The resident has the courage to follow his beliefs. But if **courage** justifies one following one's **beliefs** in interaction with another, then anything goes and interaction is impossible.

Integrity demands of a professional that he act according to his beliefs as long as these beliefs are in accord with his factual knowledge. A physician does not exercise integrity when he acts on beliefs internal to himself and unconnected to his profession.

Justice demands of a professional that he not experiment on a patient on the basis of his ungrounded opinions. A professional has no right to imperil another.

Every professional owes herself and her patients a professional attitude that makes **pride** possible. This attitude is not exhibited when one takes unquestioning "pride" in one's beliefs when there is strong evidence against these beliefs. This is vanity, not pride.

Finally, the resident's belief cannot be taken from **wisdom**. Wisdom is not a set of unchanging beliefs. If it were, reason would be unrelated to wisdom, and no one could ever achieve wisdom through one's capacity to reason. The nurse and the pharmacist have the responsibility to see that the drug is not given and that another one is ordered for Carl's pain.

Dilemma 4-3, page 72   Should a noncompliant patient be punished?

Autonomy: Dan's cause-and-effect actions are unintelligible, so the standard of autonomy gives him no support. But the same holds true of his family. So autonomy must be set aside.

Freedom: If the physician's plans involved taking resources for someone more likely to be compliant, then there is a problem. If a noncompliant patient is given full-freedom, he would exercise it in a way that would make him a nonpatient. His actions would conflict with the nature of the health care system. But, in this case, the treatment the patient is given takes nothing away from anyone. And to deny him freedom entirely would make no sense.

Objectivity: There is no obvious objective reason why the patient should not receive the treatment the physician plans. If he recovers, what his objective judgments would be cannot be known. But it is reasonable to hope for the best. The patient's mother and sister have no objective reason to deny him treatment, and their wishes should be disregarded.

Self-assertion: If the patient was denied self-assertion, the outcome would be predictable and, for him, unfavorable. If his self-assertion is given all the support possible, the outcome might possibly be favorable.

Beneficence: The benefits to the patient's relatives, whatever they might be, are completely irrelevant. There ought to be a much more significant reason for denying beneficence to a patient in the health are setting.

Fidelity: Obviously, the patient's relatives feel no fidelity to his best interest. The patient may not either. But a decision should not be made through rationalizing over what is not known.

Dilemma 5-1, page 85   Is the use of "compassionate deception" to sustain a patient's pride justified?

First off, Dee did not tell Anna, "Everyone does this." Anna's right to be different ought to be explicitly recognized. It was.

Dee accepted Anna's autonomy and she resolved the dilemma through 'indirection'. Dee asked Anna, as a favor, to taste a batch of pigs-in-the-blanket that she had made. She told Anna that she made them for her in-laws and she wanted them to be perfect. She induced Anna to try them and give her suggestions on how she might improve them. She told Anna that she had made several unsuccessful tries and asked Anna to show her how they are made. She brought the makings to Anna's home—enough so that Anna had to freeze some.

The message that Dee delivered to Anna was unmistakable: "Anna, after all the nice things I have done for you, how can you refuse to do this for me?" The dam was broken. Anna assented with some degree of joy and gratitude, knowing full well that Dee's actions had been a ploy. They shared a joke at Anna's 'expense'. Autonomy always points to the right direction. Sometimes, the direction it points to is indirection. A practice-based ethic, based on beneficence, does not require that people bump heads.

Dilemma 5-2, page 87   **Should a dying patient remain "full code" because of his family's optimism?**

Autonomy: If the desires of Edgar's family are given priority, his autonomy is obviously violated, since his desires and theirs contradict each other.

Freedom: Not to honor Edgar's wishes is obviously a violation of his freedom. The more so since there is no possibility of his achieving freedom in the future.

Objectivity: The family's optimism is a subjective feeling in conflict with the facts. Subjective feelings, except those of a patient, have no weight in a practice-based ethic.

Self-assertion: Assertion of one's values for another is not an ethical standard.

Beneficence: It is not justifiable to take over a patient's right to self-assertion in order to indulge a formalistic and malevolent whim. It is not justifiable to take over a patient's right to self-assertion in order to indulge a formalistic and benevolent whim. It is not justifiable to violate a patient's right to self-assertion for any reason. No motivation can justify this.

Fidelity: The physician's agreement with Edgar was not to act as his agent unless his family felt an optimism that he did not share.

Dilemma 5-3, page 90   **Should a dietitian provide TPN to a dying man against her better judgment because it is what the physician wants?**

Autonomy: Very few people would want TPN under these circumstances. Therefore, we must conclude that it is unlikely that Luke would. We have no reason to believe that his desires would be different from the great majority of people.

Freedom: We do not enhance Luke's freedom by giving him the freedom to suffer.

Objectivity: The physician has an ethical obligation to those he asks to assist him, in this case, Betty and the nurse. His obligation is to provide some objective reasoning in support of this course of action.

Self-assertion: We have no reason to believe that Luke would act to do this for himself. Therefore, we have no justification for doing this for him.

Beneficence: To prolong a patient's painful dying process is not beneficent. If it were, there would be no such thing as a maleficent course of action.

Fidelity: Many times, when we give fidelity to our powerful enthusiasm, we practice a fidelity to ourselves and our feeling of own "well-being." We never have a right to choose our enthusiasm over the welfare of our patient.

Dilemma 5-4, page 92   A dilemma involving a nurse's promise of secrecy.

This is not a dilemma that a nurse is very apt to find. However, the dilemma presented in this extreme case points up the principles involved in any dilemmas of this kind.

Autonomy: The patient is unique. The nature of his desire is determined by this uniqueness. How his desire is shaped by his uniqueness in the situation cannot be known. The nurse must go on the knowledge she has. But the dilemma assumes that she has very little knowledge.

Freedom: If she reveals what her patient has told her, she will, at least apparently, be taking action against him.

If she informs the physician, she will also be taking an action for him. She will be helping him to continue acting on the purpose he had in entering the hospital. The standard of freedom offers little help one way or the other. Or, rather, it offers too much help. It offers help in both directions.

Objectivity: In order to meet the demands of the standard of objectivity, a nurse must be guided by beneficence. Does objectivity call for her to keep her promise to the patient? Or does it call for her to inform the physician so that he can take the best possible action? In order to discover the demands of beneficence, she has to know the probable outcomes of different courses of action given her patient's ultimate purposes.

There is no way the nurse can know what direction beneficence takes. But all of this takes place in a health care setting, and when there is any doubt, the nature of the health care setting must determine action. Unless there are very unusual and obvious circumstances, as a rule of thumb, if the known circumstances could not outline the script for a plausible 1-hour hospital TV drama, the nurse should inform the physician.

Self-assertion: Finally, we find some assistance in the standard of self-assertion.

The nurse does not take over the ownership of her patient unless she does something for him that he would not do for himself. If she does something for him that he would do, then she is simply acting as his agent.

In considering the dilemma from the vantage point of self-assertion, it is possible to see one important fact: Silence maintains the patient's self-assertion and self-ownership only if he would be willing to harm himself.

Perhaps he would. Perhaps his reason for wanting to keep his condition secret is important enough that he would be willing to endure this harm. The nurse must ask herself, however, why he would have told her if this is the case? If secrecy here is important enough for him to endanger himself in this situation, why would he have told his nurse? Consideration of the case under the standard of self-assertion tends to indicate that the nurse should tell the physician what the patient told her.

Beneficence: Contextually, it seems as if beneficence calls for telling. But the harm of telling is not known. Action is behavior arising from knowledge. An agent should always prefer to act on what he does know rather than on what he does not know.

The harm of not telling is known. If this harm is at all serious, then that which is known must override that which is not known.

Beneficence, guided by reason, suggests that the nurse break her promise of secrecy.

Fidelity: Fidelity requires the nurse to make a choice. She must exercise fidelity either toward her promise or toward her patient. Her promise, of course, was a promise to her patient. All the same, she owes fidelity not to one aspect of her relationship to her patient, but to the entire relationship and to the destiny of her patient. In the context of a purposive ethic, she owes fidelity to her patient and **to what she knows.**

A ritualistic ethic would demand that a nurse keep her promise, but very few nurses would. A purposive ethic would demand that a nurse keep her attention on the purpose that brought her patient into the hospital.

When a patient tells a secret to a nurse, he should not forget that the first purpose of the health care system is his health and well-being. Secrecy for the sake of secrecy must give way to health and well-being.

Dilemma 5-5, page 93 Is it ever right to tell lies from benevolent motives?

Autonomy: Whatever the nature of their autonomy, it is inconceivable that Robin's parents would take a calm and disinterested view of Robin's death.

Freedom: Obviously, the power of Robin's parents to move into the future was truncated by the nurse's actions.

Objectivity: When Robin's parents heard the details of their daughter's death, this did them no good and could not fail to do them harm. It did nothing to help them assimilate this event into their lives and to begin to move on.

Self-assertion: No one's agency was increased by this. The experience they underwent at the hands of Robin's nurse will, predictably, interfere with Robin's parents getting on with their lives. They will always carry this picture in their mind.

Beneficence: Robin's nurse harmed the parents emotionally and forever. It did nothing to increase their ability to reason. Robin's nurse acted dutifully, but she failed to act beneficently. She did not fail to act irrationally.

Fidelity: Obviously, no rational purpose was served by this action. The nurse cannot justify her action by appealing to fidelity.

Dilemma 5-6, page 96   Should heroic measures be used when a terminally ill patient stops breathing?

This is clearly and easily resolved by analysis through extremes (the topic of chapter 6).

It may be that the family has Ruth's best interest at heart. They may sincerely want to do what is best for her—although the rarity of their visits would not seem to bear this out.

Freedom: Even if they are well-intentioned, the course of action they propose is precisely the same as an implacable enemy of Ruth's might propose. Because human suffering is real, undesirable, and contrary to the purpose of the health care setting, it is better that the family have no freedom in deciding on Ruth's destiny, rather than full freedom, for there is no way to know how much suffering Ruth would have to endure before they would be willing to back away from their position. On the other hand, if they exercise no freedom, this will be in line with Ruth's freedom.

Objectivity: It is better that their opinion is considered nonobjective rather than objective. For Ruth is obviously in a better position to know what is best for herself than her family.

Self-assertion: The self-assertion they would be able to control at the infrequent times when they visit is not enough to meet Ruth's needs. It is better that they exercise no surrogate self-assertion in relation to Ruth's situation.

Beneficence: Whatever their motivation, there is no reason to believe that it is a form of beneficence, and it is better for them to have no control over Ruth's benefit than full control, which is unthinkable.

Fidelity: There is no reason to believe that they feel interest in and fidelity for Ruth and her welfare. And, without fidelity, there is no justification for their having control.

Dilemma 5-7, page 97   The right of a patient to act against the belief of her culture.

Autonomy: There has been a change in Maria from the unique person she once was to the person she now is—a person whose unique character-structures have, to a significant extent, been lost. She does retain one aspect of her autonomy. She disagrees with some of the beliefs of her culture.

Freedom: Maria's freedom, her ability to take long-term actions in pursuit of her values, to a significant extent, has been lost. Maria's actions now are very much bound up with fighting her depression and anxiety. One thing has not been lost: Her right to pursue her chosen method of treatment.

Objectivity: Maria's objective awareness, and her consequent ability to deal with the facts of her circumstances, has become radically impaired. Maria's attention is now very much directed onto and shaped by her depression and anxiety. However, there is no reason to believe that her desire for treatment has been shaped by these two elements.

Self-assertion: Maria's control of her time and effort has been lost. Her time and effort is no longer directed to fulfilling her needs and values. It has been lost to her anxiety and depression. But not entirely lost. It is not necessary to take it away from her entirely in order to enable her to regain it.

Beneficence: Maria's self-seeking has been impaired. She is significantly unable to act in her own best interest. The unique person Maria was is no longer. Her self-seeking has been impaired because her self has been impaired. Her right and ability to trade has not been lost.

Fidelity: Maria is no longer able to act with fidelity to her life and values. Her psychological state has robbed her of fidelity to herself, except in regard to her desire to regain her health.

The resolution is a simple one—give Maria what she wants: care from professionals. Maria must determine for herself what she will and will not apply to herself from the belief of her culture. Otherwise, her culture is in control—it rules her and, therefore, negates her (the problem with cultural relativism).

Maria may decide, for the sake of her husband, to see the currendera, but whether she does is no part of a biomedical responsibility.

Dilemma 5-8, page 100   Should heroic measures be used to keep a dying patient who is in excruciating pain alive?

Autonomy: If heroic measures are not taken and Martha is allowed to die, then, certainly, her uniqueness will be lost along with her life. Her uniqueness will pass out of existence. This fact, however, has no ethical relevance. The ethical concept of autonomy is not the uniqueness of a person that the outside world gazes upon. It is the uniqueness of a person as the person lives and experiences it. It is the person's self-identity as he or she experiences it. Not to allow Martha to die would not preserve her autonomy. It would violate her autonomy. Not to allow Martha to die is not the same as forcing her to live. It is forcing her to continue dying.

Freedom: If it is Martha's desire to die, and health care professionals have agreed to act as her agent, then in applying heroic measures, they violate their agreement. They take an action for her that she would not take for herself.

Any claim that they violate her right to freedom in not applying heroic measures is one of the extreme points of ethical absurdity.

Objectivity: As far as making her decision is concerned, Martha has all the information she needs. Her excruciating pain and the fact that she is terminal provide this. The standard of objectivity does not enter into the picture beyond this. In her physical state, her body is reasoning for her.

Self-assertion: When a person makes an agreement with a health care professional, he or she makes it from the perspective of self-ownership. Martha made her agreement on this basis. If someone has a right to force Martha to live in these circumstances (for instance, a legislator who passes a law), then this person has taken over the ownership of Martha. This is true despite the fact that Martha has never given up her self-ownership.

It is absurd to say that Martha's self-ownership is not violated under these circumstances. If another person takes over control of Martha's actions, this person certainly violates her right to self-assertion.

Beneficence: In dilemmas involving passive euthanasia, different people have widely differing views as to what constitutes beneficence. It is, finally, up to every individual to determine what constitutes "doing good or at least doing no harm." What a person believes and what a person can justify are often very different things. Staying in the bioethical context, let us try to clarify the question of justification through a thought experiment:

Try to imagine that to end Martha's life and suffering would be to harm her.

Imagine that to keep her alive and suffering would be to bestow some good upon her.

Now that you have seen this in your mind's eye, let us take it one step further.

Imagine a patient, Marian, who is dying a peaceful and painless death. The technology to keep Marian alive is available, but is excruciatingly painful.

Assume that Marian ought not be kept alive under these circumstances, and then try to devise some justification for keeping Martha alive.

Is it not absurd to keep a patient in unendurable pain alive while permitting a patient who is not in pain to die?

Suppose that ethics demands that patients such as Marian, as well as patients such as Martha, be kept alive. This supposition implies that every health care setting ought to become a combination cemetery and torture chamber.

If a person can believe this, nothing more can be said. If a person can justify it bioethically, he or she will have transformed the nature of modern biomedicine—not necessarily for the better.

Fidelity: The demands of fidelity, of course, depend upon the agreement. If health care professionals agree to act as Martha's agents, and they agree to act toward her with beneficence, then they agree to act toward Martha as she would act toward herself. Martha would not act to keep herself alive. If health care professionals keep her alive in these circumstances, they break their agreement with her.

Euthanasia, even passive euthanasia as discussed in Martha's case, is a very complex and controversial subject. In order to illuminate the analysis we have made through the bioethical standards, we will analyze it through the elements.

Desire: It is inconceivable that the desire of a terminal patient in unbearable pain to continue living as long as possible could be a rational desire. The element of rational desire calls for allowing Martha to die.

Reason: To paraphrase the philosopher Benedict Spinoza: reason demands nothing contrary to nature; and nature demands nothing contrary to reason. If a person wages a war on his existence—a war that he cannot win—if he denies everything that he knows to be true, he turns his back on reason—on everything he is. Reason demands that a person accept the facts of his existence and the reality of his world. If reason demands anything, then it demands that a person accept that which he knows to be true.

For a person to accept that which he knows to be true is for him to act in harmony with his own nature. It is for him to act in harmony with the reality of the world around him. Reason and nature demand nothing less than this.

The reality of Martha's existence calls for the exercise of reason. It calls for the biomedical professionals who are her agents to exercise reason and beneficence.

Life: Martha is alive only in the sense that an irrational animal is alive. Martha is not an irrational animal. The best promise life offers her is death. If Martha's life is allowed to speak for itself, then Martha ought to be allowed to die.

Purpose: Analyzing Martha's situation from the vantage point of purpose shows that Martha ought to be allowed to die. This is not surprising. In the context of the bioethical standard, it is an ethical purpose. It is a rational purpose. And, not least, it is Martha's purpose for herself.

Agency: Every ethical agent in exercising agency should exercise it with courage and clarity of vision. If biomedical professionals are given the power to decide Martha's fate, they should decide with courage and clarity of vision. For they are her agents.

Both the bioethical standards and the elements suggest the ethical propriety of allowing Martha to die.

Dilemma 7-1, page 125   **Should a young girl be informed that her physician has discovered the condition of testicular feminization?**

Autonomy: There is no question that informing Amelia of her condition will be an assault on her self-image. There is no question that it will have negative effects on her (developing) autonomy. An analysis of the effects on Amelia's autonomy of being told of the condition reveal these reasons why she should not be told. It reveals no reasons why she should be told.

Freedom: It is certainly the case that Amelia will enjoy less freedom by knowing of her condition. Thus, at best, the standard of freedom does not support informing her of her condition.

Objectivity: It is hard to see how Amelia would be better off knowing of her condition. Benevolence does not call for her to be informed. The effect that being informed will have on her autonomy is an excellent reason for her not to be informed. The standard of objectivity does not justify informing her.

Self-assertion: The act of informing her would surely be an invasion of Amelia's self-assertion. She has not invited, and it is probable that she would not invite, Dr. Richmond to inform her.

Beneficence: There is no question that not informing her is the more beneficent course of action.

Fidelity: The agreement between a patient and a health care professional is an agreement that the health care professional will try to make a patient's state of well-being better and not worse.

What Dr. Richmond can do immediately will make Amelia's state of well-being better, although Dr. Richmond is not the only surgeon in the world who can do this.

On the other hand, the long-term detriment of being informed will vastly outweigh the benefit that Dr. Richmond will bestow on Amelia through his immediate action. Once Dr. Richmond does this harm to Amelia, there will be no one who can undo it.

Despite the bioethical standards, many contemporary ethicists would call for Amelia to be told of her condition. Because of the complexity of this situation, let us examine it in terms of the elements of Amelia's autonomy. (The complexity of this case makes it desirable to call on them here.)

Desire: Most 17-year-old girls would not want to be informed. It cannot be known with certainty whether Amelia would want to be informed, but it can be known with certainty that she probably would not.

Reason: Knowing of her condition will make it more difficult for Amelia to think positively of herself and her life. The element of reason calls for Amelia not to be told. Knowing would do Amelia more harm than good. There is, at least, a slight suggestion, in reason, that she not be told. If reason is to be beneficent, then there is a powerful demand that she not be told.

Life: No part of her life is threatened by not knowing. Therefore, there is nothing at all in the element of life to suggest that she should be told.

Purpose: None of Amelia's purposes would be served by her being informed. At the same time, it cannot be doubted that some of her purposes would be hindered by her knowing. The element of purpose counsels that she not be told.

Agency: Amelia's agency would be hindered by her knowing. Her self-image would be damaged. Her approach to the world would change.

Amelia has a right to know. She also has a right not to know. She has a right not to be harmed.

Contemporary ethicists offer two arguments as to why Amelia should be told:

1.   Amelia will probably find out anyway.

This is a contextual factor that must be taken into consideration in an actual context. It is, however, a factor that can be taken into consideration only in an actual, real-life context. It is a logistical factor and, as such, it is not one of the ethical aspects of the context. If there is any way that it can be brought about that Amelia will not find out about her condition, then this way should be discovered.

That Amelia will find out anyway is a rationalization. It is a health care professional's excuse for doing his duty when he knows he should not.

2.   It is suggested that Dr. Richmond has a responsibility to Amelia's relatives. Amelia must be informed in order that she can discuss this condition with them. It might be advantageous to them to be aware of the recessive disorder that may run in their family.

Let us examine the ethical strength of this argument.

Dr. Richmond may believe that he has a duty to inform Amelia's relatives. As we have seen, duty is an entirely inappropriate bioethical standard, so he cannot justifiably act on this feeling. Perhaps, however, Dr. Richmond reasons that Amelia has a duty to inform the members of her family.

There is no reason to believe that Amelia has any such duty. Claiming that Amelia has a brother (and she may have a brother) does not **prove** that she has a brother. Claiming that Amelia has a duty does not, logically or ethically, establish the fact that indeed she does have a duty. Every bioethical standard implies that she does not.

It is probable that Dr. Richmond's reasoning, strictly speaking, is not deontological. It is not based on a declaration that either he or Amelia has a duty. His reasoning, probably, is, at least partly, utilitarian. He is probably motivated by the belief that, by informing Amelia, "the greatest good for the greatest number" will be served. But it can be seen that this too involves a duty. We have also seen that utilitarianism is as inappropriate to a biomedical context as is deontology. The utilitarian standard will also fail to justify Dr. Richmond's action.

The difference, in this context, between a symphonological ethic and utilitarianism is this: According to a symphonological ethic, Amelia is at the center of the ethical context. Dr. Richmond must expect nothing of Amelia but that she pursue her own welfare and the welfare of those whom she values.

Utilitarianism, on the other hand, allows Dr. Richmond to expect Amelia to pursue the welfare of the larger number of people whether or not she values them. This simply because they are the large number. Her well-being must be sacrificed to their benefit.

If Dr. Richmond were motivated by a symphonological ethic, he would choose among contextual alternatives. Then he would decide according to rights and responsibilities. He would try to make his decision intelligible in relation to cause and effect. He would try to bring about ethical proportion and balance.

Such a decision would call for Amelia to take on the burden of knowing about her condition only if she chose to do this. If Amelia knew all the facts, she might, out of beneficence, wish to inform her relatives. Let us subject Dr. Richmond's position, under a symphonological ethic, to a rational ethical analysis.

Amelia should value her relatives only if she has some rational reason to value them. For instance, if they are abusive or contemptuous of her, she lacks a rational reason to value them. If she values them in spite of this, she has no ethical reward to offer those who are not abusive or contemptuous of her.

Amelia should choose in favor of her relatives only if she has a rational and objective reason to value them. This reason would have to be sufficient to make her willing to bear the burden of knowing of her condition. She has this objective reason only if her relatives, in turn, place a high value on her.

Let us see where this leaves us.

If Amelia's relatives place a high value on her, they will be concerned with the effect of knowing about her condition on Amelia. If her relatives would be unconcerned with the effect of her knowing of her condition, then Amelia has no objective reason to value them.

If Amelia does not have an objective reason to value her relatives, then to inform her of her condition so that she can inform them is simply to sacrifice her to the greater number. To inform her, Dr. Richmond would have to assume that Amelia is, or ought to be, motivated by self-contempt.

If her relatives place a high value on Amelia, they would not want her to undergo the trauma of knowing of her condition. They would regard the detriment to Amelia as out of proportion to the benefit to themselves.

In the context of a symphonological ethic, Dr. Richmond would have to conclude that: If Amelia has no objective reason to value her relatives, then, in the context of a symphonological ethic, beneficence will not be a rational motivation for her to be informed.

If Amelia does have objective reasons to value her relatives, then her relatives will not want Amelia to know of her condition. Their balanced and proportioned desire would not be to place Amelia's benefit above theirs. Rather, they would consider Amelia's benefit to be of greater benefit to them.

Amelia's relatives have reason to value Amelia only if she respects their desires. If Amelia respects their desires, then she ought to accede to their desires for her welfare to be protected.

It is not difficult to understand that Amelia's increased happiness and self-confidence throughout her life would be more prized by her relatives than their increased convenience.

Suppose that one of Amelia's relatives is a nurse. Should a nurse place this high a value on her convenience? How would she relate to her patients? Could you, as a nurse, place a high value on this nurse?

In the context of a symphonological ethic, there are no ethical circumstances calling for Amelia to be informed of her condition.

Nurses and the Physician's Dilemma

This is a dilemma that falls on a physician to resolve, and not on a nurse. However, in the health care system, very often a physician resolves a dilemma, but a nurse must deal with his resolution. Quite often, it is a nurse who must explain the physician's resolution to the patient and, perhaps, spend the better part of a day with the patient and/or the patient's family answering questions. These situations can be very frustrating for nurses.

Nurses should be able to analyze even the most difficult dilemmas. Knowing how to analyze difficult ethical dilemmas makes it easier to analyze simple dilemmas. It might also enable a nurse to win the respect of her colleagues in the health care system. It might make it possible for her to negotiate with them and, one hopes, to become involved with them in the decision-making process.

The implication of Dr. Richmond's duty is that his satisfaction at feeling right, which lasts for 1 hour, is of greater overall importance than Amelia's feeling of being wrong, which lasts for 60 years. This implies that, in Dr. Richmond's ethical world, he lives there all alone.

Dilemma 7-2, page 127 **Does a terminally ill patient have a right to expect something from a nurse that might be injurious to his health?**

This is several dilemmas in one:

- Whether a patient in these circumstances has the right to something he wants if it may be injurious to his health.
- Whether a physician is justified in refusing him.
- Whether a nurse has a right to disobey the physician's orders.
- Whether a nurse has an ethical agent obligation that overrides the physician's order.

Obviously, a dilemma of this complexity can be resolved only in the context. But analysis will reveal something about it.

Autonomy: Rodney's autonomy is expressed in this desire. This desire is very short-range. But, in fact, Rodney has no long-range desires. His desire is the expression of his autonomy in his present circumstances.

Freedom: If it is probable that the drink of water would not increase Rodney's suffering, or if his increased suffering could be alleviated, then we must consider the following:

When Rodney entered the health care system, he was better able to act for himself. As time passed, he sank into a more helpless state. To refuse Rodney's dying request while he is in this state is to violate his right to freedom. Had Rodney known that he would be subjected to this violation, it is, in principle, possible that he would not have come into the health care system. In light of the fact that Rodney cannot recover, the physician's action is an action entirely lacking ethical balance and proportion. It was a callous violation of Rodney's freedom.

If it is probable that the drink of water would increase Rodney's suffering, and if his increased suffering could not be alleviated, then the violation of Rodney's freedom is not outside of the agreement between Rodney and the professionals in the health care setting.

Objectivity: Julia owes Rodney an explanation of what might happen if he does take the water.

Self-assertion: Julia has a responsibility to the physician. She enjoys a position of trust in relation to the physician. It would be understandable if she did not find the position particularly enjoyable in this situation.

Julia has an agreement with her patient. If there is a low probability that the water will increase Rodney's suffering, then in failing to give him water Julia would be failing to act as her patient's agent. This would be a violation of the nurse/patient agreement and of Rodney's self-ownership.

If there is a high probability that the water will increase Rodney's suffering, then in not giving him the drink of water, Julia would not violate his self-ownership. Beneficence is one of the terms of the agreement. The agreement is an agreement to spare Rodney from suffering.

Beneficence: What is and what is not beneficent at every step of the way must be determined in the context.

Fidelity: Julia is Rodney's agent. She is also an agent of Rodney's agent—the physician. If the drink of water would increase Rodney's suffering, then Julia really does not face a dilemma. If it would not, then she must determine where her greater loyalty ought to lie. She must also decide what she is willing to risk. On the one hand, she risks retribution from the physician. On the other hand, she risks committing a senselessly cruel act.

Dilemma 8-1, page 133   Should an individual with dementia be medicated against his will to make him "easier to handle"?

Fred is aggressive, and no one has a right to be aggressive. Therefore, this is not a right that a nurse, acting as Fred's agent, must protect. Nonetheless, an attempt should be made to reason with Fred at a very basic level. This could be done somewhat as follows:

"Fred, you are not insane. You are not even stupid. Taking this medicine does not mean that you are insane. Insane people eat eggs. Insane people take aspirin. Is this a reason for you not to eat eggs or take aspirin? When you take this medicine, you feel better and live better. Isn't that the only thing that is important?" If this does not succeed, then the antidepressant ought to be given to Fred by whatever means are possible, but the less invasive, the better.

The motivation for giving Fred the medicine is not utilitarian. It is simply to protect the rights of the people who have to deal with him. Analysis by extremes quickly shows that this is the right thing to do. For instance, it is obvious that it is better that Fred should have no right to aggress than an unlimited right to aggress.

Dilemma 8-2, page 134   Is a health care professional right in attempting to compel a patient to make decisions regarding his treatment?

- It is true that, in delegating responsibility to the health care professional, a patient is exercising his freedom. The health care professional is an agent acting for his patient.
- In a health care setting, a patient's power of choice and decision are weakened. The knowledge he might act on is limited. The most rational exercise of his freedom might well be to delegate responsibility to a health care professional. This is constantly assumed in emergency situations. In these situations, the health care professional goes about his task with no questions asked.
- A patient's relationship to a health care professional, or any type of professional, does always involve a delegation of responsibility.

On the other hand,

- In delegating his right to freedom, the patient is not refusing to exercise it.
- In recognizing the nature of his autonomy, the patient is not abandoning it.
- It is ethically desirable that a patient assume responsibility for himself and delegate as little as possible. But what is as little as possible for one person in one context will not be as little as possible for another person in another context.

Dilemma 8-3, page 135   Should a dying patient be told of his condition if the information will terrify him?

Ken and Rachel are friends. Nonetheless, Rachel does not know which alternative—knowing or not knowing—Ken would choose, and she cannot directly ask him. This adds a complication to the dilemma. Because of this complication, the best way to analyze the dilemma is through the elements rather than through the standards.

The dilemma arose because Rachel is unsure of how to interact with Ken in this situation. She must analyze the elements of his autonomy as they function in this context.

Desire: Ken would desire to get his affairs in order, but he does not want to be made aware of the seriousness of his condition.

If Rachel is noncommittal (by noncommittal, we mean Rachel should say something like, "If you do not recover . . . " rather than, "Ken, you are dying and therefore . . . ") with Ken, it allows him to either deny the seriousness of his condition, or accept it internally but without having it thrust at him from the outside.

If Ken cannot be motivated in this way to get his affairs in order, then his desire is obvious. Ken, above all, does not want to know the seriousness of his condition.

Reason: A noncommittal approach on the part of Rachel can help Ken exercise his reason much better than can Rachel's thrusting the details of his condition at him.

Life: Only Ken can compute the importance of his terror in the present, as opposed to his desires for the future.

Purpose: Ken's purposes are in conflict. No one but Ken can tip the balance.

Agency: His agency is involved in getting his affairs in order. His condition precludes agency. As a long-term factor, the element of agency cannot enter into Rachel's deliberations. But, in the time left to Ken, Rachel's responsibility is to strengthen Ken's agency, to do for him what he would do for himself if he were able.

Dilemma 8-4, page 136   What is to be done when intrafamily coercion is suspected?

Autonomy: Their relationship is unique. It is uniquely complex and troubled. It will not be a simple matter for the biomedical team to adequately evaluate their relationship and advise them. Two unique personalities interacting together produce a state of affairs much more complex than a single individual. Out-of-context moralizing should be avoided.

Freedom: Ron and his mother both have a right to freely arrive at a decision and act on that decision.

Objectivity: The consultation between Mrs. Raymond and the biomedical professionals ought to go into exhaustive detail. Mrs. Raymond, quite probably, has a long time to live. Ron's future is very uncertain at best. Ron is trying to preserve his life. He cannot be faulted for this. At the same time, Mrs. Raymond's reasons for donating her kidney may not be well thought out. Her questions should be elaborated on until she has related the new information given to her to the entire context of her knowledge and the situation.

Self-assertion: No attempt should be made to interfere with Mrs. Raymond's exercise of her time and effort in donating her kidney to Ron. Every effort should be made to enable her to make a decision that reflects her actual values.

Beneficence: No one owes Ron any specific beneficence beyond performing the operation and advising him on a health regimen. No one owes him assistance in deception. Mrs. Raymond is owed the beneficence of clarity of vision. She deserves to know what she is doing. The biomedical team can help her gain this clarity of vision. She also deserves to know why she is doing what she is doing. This knowledge she must gain for herself and from herself. Skill on the part of the biomedical team might help her in this.

Fidelity: Biomedical care comes in various forms and degrees of excellence. Hopefully, fidelity toward the Raymonds will possess a high degree of excellence.

Dilemma 8-5, page 139   Should a comatose Jehovah's Witness be given a blood transfusion?

Autonomy: There is no way to have certain knowledge of this patient's autonomy.

Freedom: As his agent, his nurse ensures his freedom by acting for him. But she has no way of knowing what actions he would take if he were free, that is, if he were conscious. The fact that this patient belongs to a particular religious sect does not necessarily mean that he accepts every practice of this religion.

If he were conscious and declared that he did not want a transfusion, then, in the context of the bioethical standards, that would end it. But he is not conscious, and the direction that his freedom would take if he were is not known.

Objectivity: The standard of objectivity offers no guidance in this case.

Self-assertion: The patient is unable to express his ideas and desires. Therefore, there is no way to know what his self-assertion would consist in.

Beneficence: It is impossible to know what would be beneficent in relation to this patient.

Fidelity: This situation offers no grounds for an agreement.

This is a case a biomedical professional must decide for herself without any help from the bioethical standards. Because the nature of this patient's autonomy also is not known, the elements of autonomy offer little guidance. The decision would need to be made on the basis of the commonalities that all humans share.

The element of life offers what may be little more than a suggestion: A person's religion is, to a greater or lesser extent, an important part of his life.

But every whole is greater than any one of its parts. The patient's life is more than his religion. The best decision that can be made in this situation is that he be given the blood transfusion. This option will allow him to pursue his autonomous purposes for his life. Otherwise he will die, and all the options of his life will be closed off.

Dilemma 8-6, page 139   How does a nurse deal with a patient who makes demands on her that interfere with her attention to other patients?

The center of Irene's attention cannot be Henry alone; she has other patients. She cannot make an agreement with Henry that would violate the well-being of her other patients. Therefore, her dilemma cannot be resolved by analysis through the standards or the elements. Irene must analyze this as a triage situation.

Dilemma 8-7, page 140   A parent's right to know versus the right of a child to have his parents not know.

This is a very simple dilemma. It is resolved by the fact that Marilyn has an agreement with Bobby.

Marilyn, of course, also has an agreement with Bobby's parents. But Marilyn is a nurse. A nurse is a professional. As a professional, Marilyn's agreement with Bobby is superior to any agreement she may have with his parents. This agreement overrides any pleasure Marilyn might derive from unguarded small talk.

Many times it will happen that Bobby's health and well-being will require that his parents be given certain information. In that case, Marilyn should give them the information. But this is not because of her agreement with Bobby's parents. It is because of her agreement with Bobby.

Let us assume, for the sake of argument, that Bobby's parents have a right to know of his bedwetting. Even in this (questionable) case, they have no right to expect Marilyn to tell them. Marilyn's only responsibility in this case is to Bobby. Their knowing will not increase Bobby's health or well-being. Bobby desires Marilyn not to tell his parents. In most cases, a nurse cannot know whether a patient's desire is as well-reasoned as it might be. In this context, there is no reason to believe that Bobby's is not a perfectly rational desire.

Marilyn could very well say to Bobby, "I won't tell them, Bobby. Why don't you tell them?"

This is a loaded question. Bobby may feel a greater need to defend his request than to explain it. He may give Marilyn information she needs to make a more informed assessment of the situation.

Marilyn might reply to Bobby's parents, "Bobby is a little boy in a scary situation. Why don't you take some comfort to Bobby?" This is also a loaded question, based on the fact that if Bobby's parents are motivated by factors they are unwilling to reveal, they will probably respond with "righteous indignation" and reveal information that Marilyn ought to have. If they agree without indignation, the problem is probably solved.

Somewhere along the way, this course of action should reveal if Bobby has a problem he should not have.

Dilemma 8-8, page 141   Should a nurse give out information on the phone if this information might help or might harm her patient's best interest?

Lotte's only responsibility is to Ray. Her only agreement is with Ray. This agreement does not include taking the word of a caller and informing the caller of Ray's condition. It might seem as if Lotte is interfering with Ray's freedom. She is not. Ethically, Lotte cannot interfere with Ray's freedom unless he expresses a desire.

It is reasonable to assume that if Ray had expected a call, or regarded it as important, he would have expressed a desire to her. He would have asked her to give the caller the information he wanted. It is also reasonable to assume that, if the matter was important, the lawyer would have sent someone to the hospital. Lotte has no responsibility to assist Ray's lawyer in his failing to act as Ray's agent.

Before she gives any information to the caller, Lotte ought to talk to Ray.

Ray might be unable to talk to her. If Ray were unable to talk to Lotte, then he would be unable to talk to his lawyer.

Perhaps the caller is Ray's lawyer. In this case, it would have been better had Lotte given him the information. But Lotte could not know this. She can only justify acting on what she does know. In this context, Lotte took the only justifiable action she could.

If she gave him the information, she would have done the best thing for Ray. But she would have done the best thing by accident. It is not possible to justify an accident.

Dilemma 8-9, page 141   Should a feeble and elderly patient be let out of restraints to freely walk around?

Every possible consideration should be given to Margaret. Let us grant this without argument.

There are two different facts in conflict with each other:

1. Sandra should not assist Margaret in actions that will predictably injure her. To do this would be contrary to the nature and purpose of the health care system.
2. Aside from this, Margaret has a right to freedom of action.

These two facts can be brought into harmony if Margaret is allowed to walk around when she can be watched and assisted. When she cannot be, "gentle coercion" (persuasion) should be exerted to keep her in the safety of her wheelchair.

Sometimes a dilemma can be resolved by not choosing one possibility over another. An agent can meet both demands of the dilemma. He can do two things at different times and according to changes in the context.

Dilemma 8-10, page 142   Should a nurse interfere with a patient's activities if these activities threaten his well-being?

Autonomy: Charlie cannot leave his identity and his life situation behind.

Freedom: Ingrid deals with one aspect of Charlie's life. He deals with every aspect of his life. He has a right to be free to do this.

Objectivity: The standard of objectivity will extend as far as gentle coercion but no further. Once Ingrid has related the facts to Charlie, he has a right to do whatever he wants to do.

Self-assertion: Ingrid ought to warn Charlie. If it is possible, she should exert gentle coercion. But Charlie is a private individual and he has a right to decide and act for himself.

Beneficence: Strictly speaking, for Ingrid to do nothing is neither beneficence nor a failure of beneficence. If she interferes, this is against Charlie's freedom. Actions she takes against Charlie's freedom are not acts of beneficence. Beneficence is central here.

Fidelity: Fidelity to their agreement requires Ingrid to look after Charlie's health and well-being without violating the bioethical standards. The bioethical standards are the terms of their agreement.

Dilemma 8-11, page 143   Should a nurse give sensitive information to a family member before she has discussed this with her patient?

Karen and her nurse have an agreement. The bioethical standards are the terms of this agreement. The agreement provides Karen's nurse with no preexisting knowledge of what she ought to do in this situation.

Let us see if we can analyze the situation in terms of the elements of autonomy.

Desire: Only Karen knows what she desires. So this is no help to Karen's nurse.

Reason: It is up to Karen's reason to deal with this. Her nurse's only obligation is not to make it more difficult for Karen.

Life: It is up to Karen to integrate this situation into her life. Obviously, her nurse cannot help her with this.

Purpose: Karen's nurse has no purpose to serve and no right to try to guess Karen's purpose.

Agency: Karen's nurse cannot act as her agent in this situation.

The elements of autonomy provide no more direct guidance in this circumstance than the bioethical standards. The elements, however, do imply a principle by which the dilemma can be resolved. This principle calls for Karen's nurse to evade the question and get away. We will now turn to that principle.

Awareness and Ethical Action

Contextual action is action taken on the basis of objective judgment. Contextual action requires an awareness of the context of the situation. It also involves an agent's awareness of the context of his or her knowledge.

Awareness is not simply desirable for effective ethical action. It is absolutely essential to it.

In circumstances like that of Karen and Steve, we would suggest to the reader this overarching ethical principle:

If you do not know why you are going to do what you are going to do, do not do it.

This principle is not always easy to apply. It must be applied in a context according to the nature of the context. But it is directly implied by the elements of an ethical agent's autonomy.

Desire: An agent can be motivated by either his or her own desire or that of a beneficiary to whom the agent is responsible. If, on the other hand, an agent is aware of no desire, then the agent has no basis for action and no responsibility to act.

Reason: Not to act when one does not know what one is doing is the essence of practical reason.

Life: When you do not know why you are doing what you are doing, you cannot effectively guide your actions. You cannot know what effect it will have on your life or the life of your beneficiary. Under these circumstances, it is irresponsible to take action.

Purpose: To act without knowing what you are doing is to act purposelessly. This cannot be justified. The purpose of an action is its ethical justification.

Agency: To act without knowing what you are doing is to act without agency. It is not acting at all. It is a behavior that is not guided by awareness. It is a violation of your agency.

Dilemma 8-12, page 144   Should a nurse tell a patient's wife that a symbolic agreement the patient and family member had was not realized?

Of course, not telling Denise does not violate the standard of objectivity.

If there is any dilemma whose resolution is given right along with the context, this is it. Only a formalism utterly inappropriate to nursing would counsel Lucy to inform Denise that she had not succeeded.

We can be quite certain that Lucy would not do this.

Dilemma 8-13, page 145   A conflict between what a family needs to know and what a patient does not want his family to know.

This dilemma does not involve the relationship between Ike and Joan. The dilemma involved in this case involves the relationship between Joan and Helen.

There are legal entanglements to this dilemma. Joan and her colleagues might be sued by Helen if Joan does not give Helen the information she needs to get her affairs in order. This being the case, Ike has no right whatever to place Joan in jeopardy. He has no right to expect an agreement with Joan when she does not know the background facts of this agreement, when the agreement has nothing to do with the regimen of his health care, and when this agreement would place Joan at hazard.

Let us examine Joan's situation in terms of the elements.

Desire: No one would reasonably choose to pursue an occupation in which they would have no way to avoid periodic lawsuits. Ike has no logical right to assume that nursing is such an occupation. The law may be unclear in situations like this. This lack of clarity would not prevent Helen from suing Joan and the hospital.

Reason: If Joan were to keep Ike's confidence in this situation, it would be irrational on her part. It is irrational for Ike to expect this.

People in the biomedical professions have no implicit agreement with a patient to expose themselves to lawsuits.

Life: Joan's life would be greatly diminished if her patient's whim could place her in jeopardy.

Purpose: Joan's purpose, as a nurse, is to provide some value for her patient. She would have no motivation for this unless she had purposes for herself. If she acceded to Ike's wishes, Joan could allow herself no long-term purposes. Her future would be, at best, entirely unpredictable.

Agency: Joan's agency, as a nurse, should be devoted to the health and well-being of her patients. What Ike asks of her has nothing to do with her role as nurse. Joan can and ought to talk to Ike, and if necessary, explain why she cannot keep his condition a secret from Helen.

Dilemma 8-14, page 145 When should a nurse report a case of suspected child abuse?

It will be seen that the elements best illuminate this dilemma.

Desire: Shawn's desire for help is rational. Doris' desire for secrecy is not.

Reason: Shawn needs Alice to help him achieve the benefit of reason. Doris is not acting on reason if Alice is right in her suspicion.

Life: Shawn has a right to a better life.

Purpose: Shawn's purpose is justifiable. Doris' is not.

Agency: Alice is Shawn's agent. (If Shawn is a battered child, a great deal of good can be done. If he is not, no great harm will be done if the investigation is done in an ethical manner.)

Dilemma 8-15, page 146 Are there limits to patient confidentiality?

Autonomy: This certainly seems a unique, even a bizarre attitude on Dan's part. If Dan will not divulge the information to his children, a health care professional ought to. How doing this might be a violation or betrayal of some aspect of Dan's character-structure is difficult or impossible to understand.

Freedom: Telling his children would be a violation of his freedom if, and only if, their knowing would interfere in some way with legitimate actions Dan wants to take. This is a question that his nurse ought to discuss with him.

Objectivity: So long as the nurse remains open to the reasons why Dan does not want his children to know of his condition, she does not fail the responsibility of objectivity. If Dan will not give his nurse a justifying reason—a reason to leave the children ignorant of information they ought to have—he violates objectivity. He has an implicit agreement with his children to act in their best interest.

He tells his nurse that there is a reason, but refuses to tell her what the reason is. He is, apparently, not willing to expose his reason to analysis. This does not relieve the nurse from a responsibility as a fellow human being to provide the children (the children's mother) with the information. (This can be done post-mortem.)

Self-assertion: It is difficult to see how telling the children the facts would compel Dan to take undesirable actions—even in the broadest sense of actions. Dan ought to offer some justification on this score.

Beneficence: The nurse has no reason to believe that telling Dan's children of their father's condition would involve a failure to provide a possible benefit or cause a possible harm to Dan.

Fidelity: The nurse/patient agreement does not call for a nurse to act on blind faith. If Dan revealed his reasons to his nurse, it could possibly harm him. But, given what we know of the matter, there is no reason to believe this.

One ought to strive not to interfere with the efficient enjoyment of the self-ownership of another. Dan has a right to self-ownership. He does not own, and he has no right to frivolously disrupt the lives—the time and effort—of his children.

Dilemma 10-1, page 168   Counseling a patient who must decide on whether to gamble on a "long shot" treatment.

This is a situation that Vladimir very well might want to discuss with his nurse. If he does, it is desirable that she understand the vital and fundamental factors influencing his decision. Vital and fundamental factors, in a purposive ethic, are ethical factors.

Here the bioethical standards are irrelevant. This is not, in its most important sense, a case of a nurse dealing with a patient. Nor is this a case of a nurse helping a patient deal with another person. This is a case of a nurse acting as a sounding board in order to help her patient think and make a decision for himself. Vladimir needs self-awareness. His nurse can help him to analyze his situation by reference to the elements of his autonomy.

Desire: Vladimir will have to decide whether his greater desire is to play again or to retain the gross motor movements of his hand. Then he must examine the strength of these desires against the probabilities of realizing each one.

Reason: Vladimir must assess the benefits and detriments of each course of action. Then he must decide on what his most reasonable course of action will be in light of his rational desires.

Life: Vladimir must try to ascertain what his overall lifestyle will be if either operation succeeds or fails. Then he must decide whether he is willing to take the risks of one course of action or be content with the results of the other course.

Purpose: In assessing all the possibilities, Vladimir will have to decide on the purposes that motivate him.

Agency: When Vladimir has made a decision, he ought to think about whether this decision really reflects his character and values.

There is no question of a nurse making the choice for a patient in a case like Vladimir's. Even if she is asked, it is obvious that she ought to refuse. But, if she is skilled, her consciousness can be a mirror in which her patient can see his ideas and values reflected.

Dilemma 10-2, page 169   Is a nurse ever justified in not following a physician's orders?

The fact that Mr. Judd cannot speak for himself, and Aaron is speaking for him, ought to lead Aaron to analyze the dilemma from the elements of autonomy. If Mr. Judd did argue for himself, he would argue from his autonomy.

Desire: Mr. Judd's life functions—even though this is desire at its lowest level—are still active. This, in and of itself, provides **some** evidence that Mr. Judd wants to live. Dr. Smalley has no reason to believe that Mr. Judd would want to be taken off food and fluids. There is, at least, some evidence against Dr. Smalley's position, and there is no evidence for it.

Reason: It is too soon to know whether pleasure or pain will prove the major factor in Mr. Judd's future. Mr. Judd could not make an objective decision for himself based on the knowledge available to him. If he cannot, certainly Dr. Smalley cannot.

Life: Mr. Judd's life has changed. Life is constantly changing. The mere fact that it is changing, when there is no way to know what direction the change will take, does not justify withdrawing food and fluids.

Purpose: Dr. Smalley proposes to take over Mr. Judd's purposes—to exercise Mr. Judd's time and effort. Dr. Smalley has no right to do this in these circumstances.

Agency: Dr. Smalley's efforts would not increase Mr. Judd's agency. They would entirely nullify it.

Aaron ought not condemn Dr. Smalley to Mr. Judd's family. But he is certainly justified in advising them against withdrawing food and fluids.

Dilemma 10-3, page 175   How a nurse deals with a young person in exceedingly difficult circumstances.

Bioethical dilemmas are among the most complex and difficult that any human being ever faces. Wally's case is certainly among these. It will be difficult to resolve this dilemma with optimum beneficence—in such a way that Wally is done some good and no harm. If she handles it badly, a nurse can do Wally much more harm than good. A nurse who can handle this beneficently must be able to exercise a sort of ethical artistry.

Autonomy: Wally is in the health care system. The health care system has its own specific structures and purposes. The health care system is responsible for the health and well-being of everyone who enters it.

On the other hand, Wally is young. He did not come into the health care system on his own. He was not even brought in after discussion. He is suddenly thrust into a strange environment.

Taking Wally for débriding without his consent suggests that Wally's body can be taken for treatment and his consciousness can be left behind. This interaction between Iris and Wally would be truly inhuman. Iris' momentary reflection on her own nature would show her that such interaction is ethically undesirable.

Whatever its benefits, and they are obvious, compelling Wally to go for treatment at this time would violate his autonomy.

Freedom: It is part of the implicit agreement that is the basis of human rights that the young shall be protected. What are the right and wrong things for Iris to do depends on the context of her relationship with Wally. It may be necessary for her to establish a rapport with Wally very quickly. There are overwhelming reasons why Wally ought to go for débriding. Nonetheless, if Iris were to take him by coercion, this would be a violation of his freedom.

Objectivity: If Iris is to deal with Wally on the basis of objectivity, she will have to tell him that his mother is dead. The absence of ethical value in this is obvious. For Iris to put both burdens on Wally at one time would be fiendish. She would increase Wally's objective awareness in a context where this would decrease Wally's ability to act on objective awareness. She would abandon her own objective awareness of the nature of the health care system and the meaning of her role in it.

Self-assertion: Wally now has some self-ownership. He has the potential for full self-ownership. Badly handled, the overwhelming adversity he faces can stunt this potential. A nurse never knows how much good or how much harm in a person's life she can do. Her pride ought to compel her to do the best she can.

Beneficence: Beneficence calls for Iris to do as much good and as little harm as possible. Ideally, this would consist in finding a way to get Wally to treatment without inflicting force on him. It would involve telling him of his mother's death under optimum circumstances.

Fidelity: The nurse/patient agreement begins with an exchange of values. This may be the best way for Iris to proceed in order to do good and avoid harm to Wally. It may be best for her to continue this exchange. Iris needs to hang loose. She needs to bargain with Wally, to find some way to trade values with him. This will avoid the trauma to Wally that a violation of his autonomy and freedom would involve.

A skillful and effective nursing intervention here calls for Iris to treat Wally not as a "big boy," but as a human person. Although Wally is legally a minor, this is a very fine place to avoid paternalism.

Analysis under the elements of Wally's autonomy might clarify even more what is to be done.

Desire: Wally's desire to wait for his mother is rational. Force is irrational. Force would be a psychological assault on Wally.

Suppose Wally had been treated at the scene of the fire. He probably could have been treated without a prior discussion and without psychological harm. But his hospital room takes him away from the noise and stress of the disaster. It suggests that now there is a chance to think and to discuss. The situation calls out for Iris to bargain with Wally.

Wally is very fortunate if Iris has the abilities of a "con-man." Iris should not tell Wally that his mother is alive. Aside from this, at this moment, truth is the last thing to be considered.

Reason: In Wally's context, it is perfectly reasonable for him to want the comfort of his mother's presence. Effective and skillful communication and trade will have to be carried out at this level. There is probably no way Wally can reason on a more abstract level than this.

Life: Wally ought to be treated with the highest consideration. With the loss of his mother, he is at a point where he must begin to build his life again.

Purpose: In order for Iris to trade with Wally effectively, she must discover the nature of Wally's most rational (practical) purposes. She must discover what she can do to make Wally see his most desirable purposes under these conditions of his life.

Agency: The purpose of exchanging values with Wally is to enlist his desire for some purpose, to motivate his agency, and to increase his cooperation with Iris.

Dilemma 10-4, page 178   Do a child's rights protect him against a procedure he does not desire?

The concept of rights is very difficult to deal with here. For purposes of bioethical analysis, rights as we have discussed is:

. . . the product of an implicit agreement among rational beings, by virtue of their rationality, not to obtain actions nor the product of actions from others except through voluntary consent, objectively gained.

1.   In the same way the rights' agreement arises, among all people every-where, another agreement arises. This agreement arises by virtue of the reasoning power of a parent, the undeveloped state of a child's reasoning power, the naturally dependent state of the child, and the bonds of love that exist between parent and child. It is the agreement that a parent will protect and nurture the child. It is a bond of benevolence uniting parent and child. This agreement calls for a parent to decide for a child in a situation where the child is incapable of deciding for himself. Sandy's mother does have a moral right to sign the consent form.

2.   Sandy's nurse has a moral right to give him the preoperative medications. She is acting as the agent of Sandy's mother. She is doing what Sandy's mother would do if she were able.

3.   The surgeon is also acting as her agent. He also is doing what Sandy's mother would do if she could.

4.   Sandy will acquire the rights that would protect him against this procedure when there is no longer a need for the parent/child agreement.

5. Sandy's mother, the surgeon, and the nurse have rights that would protect them from undergoing this procedure involuntarily. With maturity, they have acquired this right.

6. Sandy's mother, the surgeon, and the nurse acquired the rights that they possess when they acquired the experience and the rational capacity to decide for themselves.

7. Sandy will acquire the rights that his mother, the surgeon, and the nurse possess when he acquires the experience and the rational capacity to take over his parent's role in making his vital and fundamental decisions.

8. Sandy will acquire the right to decide for his children when his reason becomes more powerful than his emotions.

Sandy's desire is not a rational desire. It is the short-term whimsical desire of a child. It is true, and Sandy knows it to be true, that his desire must give way before the parent/child agreement.

Sandy's uniqueness cannot protect him. It will begin to protect him only when it becomes a rational autonomy. Until then, it is not sufficient for the exercise of rights. No irrational autonomy will protect Sandy's short-term urges only against his rational self-interest. He becomes ethically autonomous only when his autonomy is strong enough to protect Sandy against his whims.

Dilemma 10-5, page 180   **Does a physician have the right to compel a patient to undergo a procedure that she believes the patient ought to undergo, against the patient's wishes?**

Even assuming that this is a procedure that he ought to undergo, Roger's physician and the court were not justified in the course of action they took. Roger's reasoning and decision might not have been the best, but they are not entirely irrational. Sometimes, the rights of others prevent us from doing that which we very much want to do. If this were not the case, there would be no reason for the existence of rights. Roger's rights should have prevented the physician from doing what she wanted to do.

A health care professional's role cannot give him extraordinary rights. These extraordinary rights would be a right to violate the rights of others. There cannot be such a thing as a right to violate the rights of others. If there were such a right, there could not be any rights at all.

The nurse's role in this situation would be to counsel Roger, to apply "gentle coercion," and to offer no encouragement to Roger's physician.

Let us assume that the method by which the judge declared Roger incompetent became a method common in the legal system. It is obvious that this would make the legal system an all-powerful tyranny where no one would have any rights whatever. The purpose of the judicial system would no longer be to protect rights. Its purpose would be to arbitrarily establish rights for some people and to violate the rights of others. If this were permissible in this case, one would be hard pressed to establish a point at which it is no longer permissible.

There are several significant differences between Roger's situation and Sandy's:

- There is no parent/child agreement between Roger and his physician. There is no basis for such an agreement between them.
- Because of the parent/child agreement, Sandy's rights were not violated. Roger's rights were violated.
- Sandy does not have the rational capacity nor the experience to decide. Roger has. Sandy is immature. Roger is not immature or even senile.

At his age, Sandy's situation speaks for itself. Roger's does not. Sandy's mother has a right to speak for Sandy. Roger has a right to speak for himself.

Dilemma 10-6, page 192   How to "turn around" a patient who has lost hope.

Negative thoughts and emotions have overwhelmed her autonomy. The task is to overcome these negative emotions with positive ones. This can be done, if at all, through the elements of autonomy.

Desire can be used to inspire positive thought processes to increase her desire. It is important that the positive values that are possible to her—given a state of living that she can enjoy—overcome the influence of her immediate negative experience.

The elements of her autonomy, if she is to put her life back together, will strengthen her desire to act, her objective awareness, and her fidelity to the life that is still hers for the taking. Despair is best combated through the elements.

To inspire Jody to meet the challenges life presents and regain the possibilities her life offers would be a splendid ethical achievement. Nonetheless, there is a vast difference between achieving this entirely for Jody's sake and achieving it for the sake of others.

Dilemma 10-7, page 199   Should a psychiatric patient who is brought into the hospital against his will be forcibly medicated?

There is a strong tide of opinion that supports the idea that, "Every human being of adult years and sound mind has a right to determine what shall be done with his own life . . . " (President's Commission, 1982, p. 20).

Everyone has the right to be free of outside interference. The acceptance of a person's right to determine what will be done with his or her life ought to be part of the mind set of every person involved in making ethical decisions for others.

Competency is very difficult to assess. According to the President's Commission of 1982, the assessment of competency depends upon values, goals, choices, life plans, and purposes. The assessment of competency, then, is an ethical assessment. Ethics is concerned with values, goals, choices, life plans, and purposes. It is not surprising that the issue of competency makes many ethical abuses possible. The criteria for assessment that the President's Commission has set down are ethical criteria. The criteria are ethical in the framework of a symphonological ethic. The President's Commission (1982, pp. 57–60) proposed three elements of competency. To establish competency, a person must:

1.   Possess a set of values and goals that are reasonably consistent and that remain reasonably stable so that they do not radically conflict.
2.   Have the ability to understand and communicate information so that it can be known that this person can appreciate the meaning of potential alternatives.
3.   Have the ability to reason and deliberate about choices in light of values, so that he or she can compare the impact of alternative outcomes on personal goals and life plans.

A person's decision-making capacity is impaired if it fails to, at least, minimally promote his or her desires and purposes.

It is very difficult to determine incompetency. A patient who does not want to do what a nurse or physician wants him to do, or what they think is best for him to do, is not necessarily incompetent. It may be that this patient has a better outlook on the context of his life than either the nurse or physician. With this better outlook, his judgment may be superior to that of the nurse or the physician.

On the other hand, it is not necessary to regard every statement a person makes as reflecting his desires and purposes. A child's vision is not sufficiently long range to always express his real desires and purposes. The same may be true of a patient in extreme pain, one in shock, or one with brain metastasis, mental retardation, or psychiatric problems. He may be able to act, at best, only on urges. The difference between desires and purposes, on the one hand, and urges, on the other, is that the latter are short-term motivations while the former are integrated into a person's life.

The desires of the truly incompetent patient are not the result of an objective reading of the facts facing him. In this sense, they are not desires at all. The expression of his desires is the product of a type of free association.

If a person is unable to express his desires and purposes, this, in itself, does not establish that someone else has a right to do it for him. The best that another person can do is to help him establish a longer-range outlook. Ideally, a health care professional, when dealing with an incompetent patient, would ally himself with that patient as he is when he has a clear vision of his life purposes.

The situation of an incompetent patient is very much like the situation of a child, with one major difference: The child is in this situation a very long time; the patient, it is hoped, will be in this situation a very short time.

For different reasons, neither an incompetent patient nor a child has the rational capacity to make decisions. The relationship between a health care professional and an incompetent patient is the most delicate of all bioethical relationships. It may be that this relationship calls for an agreement very similar to the parent/ child agreement.

When acting for an incompetent patient, a health care professional must attempt to do for the patient what the patient would do for himself if he were able. The health care professional must try to put himself in his patient's shoes. In order to do this, he must obtain some familiarity with a patient's situation and values. If he cannot obtain this understanding of the patient's context, then perhaps he should act toward his patient as he would act toward the naked comatose stranger of chapter 10. This requires that he protect his patient against himself and other health care professionals. A health care professional can look upon the treatment of a psychiatric patient either from the perspective of utilitarianism or as a triage situation.

From the utilitarian perspective, the professional's viewpoint will be "extensionalist." He will be interested in the effect of his action on the group—on the patient's family, the rest of the hospital staff, etc. His goal will be the greater good for the greatest number, not the welfare of his patient. This cannot fail to narcotize his concern for his patient.

If he looks at the situation as though it had the same form as a triage situation, his viewpoint will be "intentionalist." He will be interested in the effect of his action on his patient. This will make the welfare of his patient the center of his attention. This is where the center of his attention belongs.

The legal and ethical positions of the incompetent patient are very often in conflict. Ideally, ethical decisions would be made for the incompetent patient only within the following parameters:

For a health care professional to assume responsibility, make ethical decisions, and take actions for a patient, there ought to be some implicit or explicit invitation for him to do so. Otherwise, there is a violation of the patient's self-ownership. With the violation of the patient's self-ownership, there is coercion. Coercion is not ethically justifiable.

The only exception to this would be in a situation strongly analogous to that of the naked, comatose stranger. But, even here, there is a kind of implicit invitation.

There are times when the psychiatric patient is in virtually the same state as the naked, comatose stranger. Then the same conditions for treatment would hold.

A radical ethical differentiation should be made between the patient who comes into the health care setting voluntarily and the patient who does not. The patient who comes in voluntarily makes an implicit agreement with the people in the health care setting. The patient who does not enter voluntarily makes no such agreement. His self-assertion is violated. If he has a right to self-assertion, he has a right to refuse to make an agreement. He has a right to have this refusal accepted.

This is the only course of ethical action consistent with the bioethical standards. This course of ethical action is very much at odds with the laws presently governing these situations. The current laws provide the patient some protection; however, they provide much more opportunity for exploitation.

There is a very old saying, to the effect that, "Where there are many laws, there is much tyranny." This is because where there are many laws, people do not concern themselves with ethical thinking or ethical analysis. They come to follow the letter of the law and, beyond this, they do whatever is convenient.

It goes without saying that this only holds when the patient has not threatened or committed any criminal action. If he has, then of course the ethics of the situation are very different.

Bioethicist Morris Abram, head of the President's Commission for the Study of Ethical Problems in Medicine and Biomedical and Behavioral Research (1982), stated:

> . . . while recognizing the important role that the law has played in this area, the Commission does not look to the law as the primary means of bringing about needed changes in attitudes and practices. Rather, the Commission sees "informed consent" as an ethical obligation that involves a process of shared decision making based upon the mutual respect and participation of patients and health professionals. Only through improved communication can we establish a firm footing for the trust that patients place in those who provide their health care. (p. 32)

Everyone, whatever his or her condition in life, possesses individual rights and ethical status. People possess rights by virtue of their rationality. This does not mean that someone who is irrational does not possess rights. The possession of rights is species wide. Everyone, regardless of physical or psychological conditions, possesses the right to ethical treatment. Suppose it were possible to pick and choose which members of the human species would have their rights recognized. Obviously, under these circumstances, there could be no trust among ethical agents.

Without the possibility of trust among ethical agents, no one could possibly possess rights. For this reason, the possession of rights must be enjoyed by every member of the species. When making a decision for an incompetent patient, it is especially important to make the decision according to the values and goals of the patient. Otherwise, the bioethical standards have been violated.

Throughout history, the treatment of psychiatric patients has been the scandal of medicine. Every health care professional ought to remain fully aware of the right of an individual to make decisions for his or her own life. When it becomes necessary to force a patient to do something or to restrain the patient from doing something, a health care professional should never take the situation as the status quo.

The difficulties of dilemmas involving psychiatric patients are very complex. They cannot be captured in a case study. In Jason's case, it certainly appears that his agency is impaired. In all likelihood, if he were in touch with his life, he would want to recover from his present condition. If it is justifiable to treat him against his expressed desires (or urges), the person who does treat him should not lose sight of the fact that the purpose of treatment is to return Jason's agency to him.

REFERENCE

President's Commission for the Study of Ethical Problems and Medicine and Biomedical and Behavioral Research. (1982). *Making health care decisions: The ethical and legal implications of informed consent in the patient-practitioner relationship* (Vol. I). Washington, DC: U.S. Government Printing Office.

Glossary

abstract   Refers to the more general and less contextual. "John" is an individual concrete. "Boy" is an abstraction. "Male" is still more abstract. "Person" more abstract still. "A nurse ought to be faithful to her agreement with every patient who comes under her care" is more abstract (more general and less contextual) than "This nurse ought to be faithful to her agreement with this patient."

acceptance   Engagement with an instrument, with one's objective knowledge, or with another agent in order to realize a purpose.

action   A behavior arising in the volition of an agent to which the agent assigns a personal meaning. A behavior that an agent initiates from within, and that remains under the agent's control.

agent   One who initiates action or one who is capable of taking internally generated action.

agency   The power or capacity of an agent to initiate action.

agreement   A propensity or formal potentiality in existents to behave in specific ways and no others when they are interacting; a shared state of awareness—a meeting of the minds—on the basis of which interaction occurs.

analysis   The process whereby one seeks to understand a whole by examining its basic parts or a process of awareness aimed at understanding.

animal For purposes of bioethical analysis, any organism capable of moving about from place to place on the power of its own agency. This obviously includes humans.

apathy Lack of interest in the things that a person generally considers worthy of attention.

appropriate Whatever gives an agent a greater power of agency is appropriate for that agent; for instance, an understanding of the nature of a dilemma is appropriate for its solution. Freedom from suffering and disability are appropriate to every human being. That which produces intelligibility in the relations between ethical causes and effects (responses); that is appropriate that increases intelligibility, supports the continuation of causal chains, and enables an agent to realize his purpose.

arbitrary A belief, conclusion, or decision is arbitrary when it is not based upon compelling evidence—when another belief, conclusion, or decision could have been chosen just as well.

autonomy As a bioethical standard, the uniqueness of every individual person. This uniqueness is the specific nature—the character-structure—of that person. One's autonomy includes his specific identity and consequent ethical equality with all other rational agents. Primarily, however it refers to an agent's uniqueness.

balance The property of an interaction whereby there is a mutual exchange of values; a satisfactory arrangement of value received for value given. Reciprocity. Balance and proportion are maintained when there is a parity between benefit given and benefit received, or harm inflicted and harm returned. Balance and proportion are lacking when a harm is returned for a benefit or vice versa. In one sense, balance and proportion are beneficence. In the same sense, they are justice. Insofar as balance involves benefit, it is beneficence.

benefactor An agent who acts so as to bring about a benefit to a beneficiary.

beneficiary One who benefits from an action. The recipient of a benefit.

beneficence "To help or at least to do no harm" (Hippocrates). The act of assisting a patient's effort to attain that which is beneficial. The desire to benefit one with whom one empathizes. As a bioethical standard, the power of a patient (or professional acting as the agent of a patient) and the necessity he faces to act to acquire the benefits he desires, and the needs his life requires.

benefit   "Something that enhances or promotes well-being" (American Heritage Dictionary, 1997).

benevolence   A psychological inclination to beneficence.

bioethics   A system of standards arising with the professional agreement to determine, sanction, and justify the interaction of biomedical professional and patient.

burn-out   "A syndrome of physical and emotional exhaustion involving the development of a negative self-concept, negative job attitude, and loss of concern and feeling for patients" (Pines and Maslach, 1978).

character-structure   Every standard taken as a virtue plays a part in structuring the individual nature of a person. Each standard, in this sense, is a character-structure. The interlocked virtues that produce and explain the individual's characteristic actions are his or her character-structure.

choice   The intentional resolution of an alternative.

coercion   The act of compelling someone, by threats or force, to act in a particular manner. The act of forcibly restraining, compelling, or controlling another person.

cognition   The act of grasping the defining or relevant properties of an object.

concept   A mental image, held in the mind, of something existing in reality; the act by which a person knows an object in reality; the idea of that which is known.

conditions   Existing circumstances. The circumstances that are necessary in order for some state-of-affairs to come about.

consequences   That which follows as the result of a cause; the moral effects of an initiated cause.

context   The interweaving of the relevant facts of a situation—the facts it is necessary to act upon to bring about a desired result and the knowledge one has of how to most effectively deal with these facts.

(*of the situation*) The interwoven aspects of a situation that are fundamental to understanding the situation and to acting effectively in it.

(*of knowledge*) An agent's awareness of the relevant aspects of a situation that are necessary to understanding the situation and to acting effectively in it.

(*solitary context*) A context involving only one person—the agent.

(*interpersonal context*) A context involving more than one person.

cultural relativism   The theory that what is ethical and what is unethical is determined by the customs, beliefs, and practices of a culture or society.

decision   A choice made between alternative values and consequent courses of actions.

deontology   "The theory that . . . actions in conformance with . . . formal rules of conduct are obligatory regardless of their results" (Angeles, 1992).

desire   One's psychological orientation toward a purpose. The capacity of an organism whereby it acts to retain its values, including the value that is its own life.

determinism   The doctrine that human choices are the effects of necessitating conditions; the theory that all conscious behavior is a response to outside forces in the same way that the behavior of physical entities is a response to external forces.

determine   To bring something—a state of awareness or a state of being—into existence; to direct a course of action.

dilemma   A situation in which one is faced with a conflict of purposes or with purposes whose value is not clear.

duty   An ethical sanction demanding adherence to a rule without regard to consequences.

element   "The fundamental, essential, or irreducible constituent of an object" (American Heritage Dictionary, 1997). Thus the roundness of a ball is an element of a ball. Its color is not.

emotivism   The doctrine that holds feelings or emotions as forms of ethical knowledge. The doctrine that every ethical judgment is a disguised description of a person's feelings.

epistemology The study of how knowledge is acquired and retained, and how truth is identified.

ethics A system of standards to motivate, determine, and justify actions (self-assertion) directed (objectivity) to the pursuit (freedom) of vital (fidelity) and fundamental (autonomy) goals (beneficence). Ethics is not convenience and it is not etiquette.

ethicist One engaged in the theoretical study of ethics.

evil The evil in relation to an ethical agent is that which negates (blocks) its efficient functioning as the kind of thing it is (failure, the violation of rights and illness are, for instance, all evils); disruption of an intelligible, causal sequence in knowledge or action; inappropriate or disproportionate to the context.

existential Concerning human existence and that which benefits human existents.

explicit Actually spoken or agreed to—not merely understood implicitly.

extremes A method of analysis through which a health care professional can clarify a bioethical context by identifying the relationships—the rights and responsibilities—of the people involved in the context.

fidelity Adherence to the terms of an agreement. As a bioethical standard, an individual's faithfulness to his autonomy. For a nurse, it is a commitment to the obligation she has accepted as part of her professional role.

flourishing The realization of human development and its potentialities (e.g., happiness); enjoying happiness based on circumstances desirable and appropriate to one's time of life.

foreseeable Predictable according to that which is given in the context.

formalism The theory that ethical action is action that conforms with certain forms of behavior; an ethical formalist is one who concentrates entirely on the abstract category into which an action can be placed, without regard for the context or the effects of the action.

freedom As a bioethical standard, self-directedness. An agent's capacity and consequent right to take independent, long-term actions based on the agent's own evaluation of a situation.

fundamental   Essential to making a thing the kind of thing it is; the fundamental element of a thing is that which best explains its behavior (for instance, roundness is essential to the rolling of a ball; therefore, roundness is a fundamental property of a ball).

gentle (as in "gentle coercion")   Simple coercion destroys a patient's ability to act on his understanding of his situation, on his notion of self-ownership, or on his conception of benefit and harm. "Gentle coercion" involves dialogue with a view to persuasion—but persuasion by means of activating, or at least not destroying, a patient's understanding and self-ownership. A form of persuasion that is neither disinterested nor an attempt to take over control of a person's time and effort. Gentle coercion does not attack a person's reasoning power. It is an appeal to that person's reasoning power.

good   The good of a thing is that which assists its efficient functioning as the kind of thing it is (i.e., success, fidelity, respect for rights, and health care are all goods); appropriate or proportionate to the context.

hedonism   The ethical theory that only those actions that produce pleasure in the agent are appropriate ethical actions.

howler   An assumption or belief that, if it were true, would have to be false. For instance, "I can be certain of nothing. . . . " If this were true, one could not be certain (know) that one can be certain of nothing.

imperfect objectivity   An imperfect objectivity is the objective awareness that one person has of the character-structures, and motivations arising from the character-structures, of another. This objectivity is indirect and mediated by factors such as introspection onto one's own character-structures.

implicit   Understood, but not as a focus of intention. Understood without being openly expressed. That of which one is not consciously aware, but which can be brought to conscious awareness.

indirection   That which characterizes bargaining with a patient in a way that avoids predictable conflict.

integrity   A virtue that characterizes an ethical agent in his fidelity to his own objective values and agreements. Fidelity to oneself.

intelligible   Structured in such a way as to be understandable.

intelligibility That aspect of an object or state of affairs whereby it is recognizable as the kind of thing it is (if the fundamental nature of a state of affairs is easily recognizable, then the state of affairs is intelligible; if any aspect of a state of affairs makes the state of affairs recognizable, then that is its fundamental aspect).

intention The state of affairs that an agent acts to bring about; a mental act of attention to an object.

interaction A chain of actions arising from agreement and interwoven in a cause and effect sequence.

interagent One who interacts.

interpersonal ethics A system of standards arising with an agreement to motivate, determine, and justify the implicit presuppositions of interaction.

interwoven Systematic; composed of interacting, interrelated, or interdependent facts that form a complex whole (e.g., sweaters are made up of interwoven strands of yarn; ethical contexts of the interweaving of circumstances and awareness).

introspection The act of directing one's attention back into one's own subjectivity; the act of reflecting back onto one's own psychological processes.

justice The concept justice can, perhaps, be best understood by analogy to a much more basic concept—the concept of physical causality. Physical objects act and interact on the basis of what their nature permits them to do—and they cannot act contrary to this. Justice, then, is to ethical agents as causality is to physical objects. Physical objects cannot interact acausally or unjustly. Ethical agents, however, have the power to choose, and they can choose either appropriately (so that, intelligible cause and effect relationships are maintained—which is justice; or in such a way that the intelligible cause and effect relationships between actions and reactions are lost—this is injustice).

justify To describe or explain in terms of, or as related to, an agreed-upon purpose.

justification A description in terms of how something meets a purpose—the purpose as formulated in a decision or agreement; demonstration that something is correspondent with the terms of an agreement.

life   The process wherein an organism generates and sustains actions directed toward the attainment of its needs and purposes according to its potential; a process whose natural product is flourishing.

logical   According to the demands of understanding; intelligible.

maleficence   To do harm or to refuse to do good where good might be expected.

meaning (in ethics)   Relation to a purpose. The meaning of **X** to an agent is the way **X** assists or hinders an agent's purpose or an agent's flourishing.

metaphysics   In the tradition—"The study of being qua being." (Aristotle in McKeon, 1941); the study of what is real in reality. For instance: That everything is what it is, that nothing is what it is not; a demonstration of why something is what it is. Or that something has a foundation in reality. For instance: Symphonology has a foundation in reality since, throughout reality, agreement produces harmony. The lack of agreement either produces nothing or produces discord.

mores   Rules or standards of behavior as related to a certain society; the ethical conventions of a society.

motivation   The reason that an agent takes an action. As the desire not to get wet is the motivation for opening one's umbrella; fear is one's motivation for taking flight; the desire to gain benefits only possible, or more easily acquired, through cooperation, is one's motivation for entering into an agreement.

native   A decision maker with the same affliction as the person for whom the decision is being made (Siegel, 1993).

necessary   It is probably not necessary to define "necessary." But if a certain state of affairs, **A**, can be an actual state of affairs only if another state of affairs, **B**, is actual, then **B** is necessary to **A**. This is the thrust of "necessary" throughout the book.

normative   "Having to do with an established standard of behavior" (Runes, 1983); having to do with ethics.

nurse (or any health care professional)   The agent of a patient, doing for the patient (given education and experience) what he would do for himself if he were able.

objective   Existing apart from a perceiving subject; having actual existence or reality; as in objective awareness: Directed outward to the characteristics necessary to establish cognition of an object.

objectivity   As a bioethical standard, a desire to know something as it is apart from emotion or personal prejudice; a patient's need to achieve and sustain the exercise of his objective awareness.

obligation   There are two products of every agreement. That which one stands to gain is the benefit of the agreement. That which one promises in return is one's obligation under the agreement.

offer   A circumstance or an object that can be known, or the state of mind of another ethical agent that seems to promise to serve a purpose if one engages with it.

passion   A behavior that an agent undergoes through a force external to self and not as the outcome of his or her act of self-determination.

patient   One who has lost or suffered a decrease in agency. One who is unable to take the actions his survival or happiness requires.

perfect agreement   An objective agreement is an agreement to interact made between two agents, when their interaction is based on an objective awareness of the circumstances influencing their interacting and its foreseeable result. A perfect ethical agreement is an objective agreement where each agent is objectively certain that the other is the right person with whom he should be interacting.

perfect objectivity   This relates to an agent's direct and immediate awareness of his own character-structures as experienced in the standards taken as his virtues. It denotes the objective awareness one has in relation to the standards as his own character-structures, values, and motivations. The differences between perfect and imperfect objectivity are fundamental.

precondition   "A condition that must exist before something else can occur" (*American Heritage Dictionary*, 1997). That which is related to something else in such a way that it is necessary to the existence of that second thing. As parents are the precondition of a child, language is a precondition of literature; objectivity is a precondition of an agreement.

presupposition   Very much like precondition, but having more to do with the context of one's knowledge. That which must be assumed if that of which it is a presupposition is assumed. Knowledge of the fact that Paul is or was a child presupposes knowledge that Paul had parents. Knowledge of the fact that a culture has produced literature presupposes knowledge of the fact that the culture possesses a language. Knowledge of the fact that one has formed an agreement presupposes knowledge of the fact that one is free to form an agreement, etc.

pride   The objective conviction that one is worthwhile.

principle   The motivating ground of an action. A basic fact, truth, or law from which other facts, truths, or laws proceed. A basic cause from which other causes arise.

professional   One who is capable, by education, training, and experience to enter a profession and to act effectively in it.

proper   Appropriate to a context; meeting a requisite standard.

proportion   A measure of benefit or value between one action or the product of the action in comparison with another action or the product of another action according to reciprocity. In one sense, balance and proportion are beneficence. In the same sense, they are justice.

purpose   That state of affairs that is the object of an action motivated by desire; the psychological condition that accompanies an orientation toward bringing about this state of affairs.

rational   Tending to appropriate proportions; well reasoned; appropriate to the context.

reason   The faculty of thinking; thinking being a process of awareness directed toward: (1) what is relevant, (2) what is appropriate, (3) what is balanced, and (4) what is proportional—in the demands of a context and the agent's responses to these demands.

reciprocity   An appropriate balance between value given and value received. A balanced interchange of benefits or values.

relevant   Necessary to the understanding of a context. Serving to bring about balance and ethical proportion (something is relevant to a context if the context cannot be fully understood without it).

responsibility The ethical link connecting an agent to the consequences of the changes he has caused to come about.

rights The product of an implicit agreement among rational beings, by virtue of their rationality, not to obtain actions or the product of actions from others except through voluntary consent, objectively gained. Rights means, in one sense, the product (freedom from aggression) of an agreement (not to aggress). In another sense, rights is the agreement itself. In either sense, the generic term (freedom from aggression; agreement) is singular. Therefore, the term rights is a singular term. It is a grave ethical mistake to regard the term rights as a political rather than a more fundamental, ethical term, and to regard it as plural—an ever-changing product of legislation.

ritualistic ethic An ethical system that holds that ethical principles are right or wrong without regard for the desires, choices, and purposes of the people involved or the consequences of ethical action.

sameness While individual things are not the same as individuals, they are the same as members of the same genus. John and Mary are merely similar to each other as individuals, as members of the genus, person, they are the same.

sanction The word "sanction" has various meanings. In ethics, it is used to mean "agreement" or "cooperation" in a broad, metaphorical sense. For instance: Criminals do not have the sanction of reason. Nature sanctions actions taken with foresight. Reality does not sanction irresponsible actions.

self-assertion The power and right of an agent to control his time and effort. It implies a person's self-ownership. As a bioethical standard, the right of an individual to be free of undesired or undesirable interaction; the right to control one's time and effort; the right to initiate one's own actions.

solitary ethics A system of standards to motivate, determine, and justify decisions and actions taken in the pursuit of an agent's own vital and fundamental goals.

standard That by which the ethical appropriateness of an action can be measured. Various standards that have been proposed are: Socrates: Knowledge of that which is beneficial; Plato: The Form of the Good; Aristotle: The actions that noble and virtuous people would take; Aquinas: Happiness; Spinoza: The preservation and enhancement of the agent's life; Kant: Duty; Bentham: The greatest good for the greatest number; Ayn Rand: The preconditions of "man's life qua man."

sufficient　One thing, **A**, is sufficient to another thing, **B**, if the existence of **A**, in and of itself, makes necessary the existence of **B**. For instance, the existence of lightning is sufficient to the existence of thunder. Thunder cannot exist without lightning. Lightning cannot exist without producing thunder. Desire is not sufficient to action—one may feel desire without acting. But action is sufficient to justify a belief in the existence of desire. Action is a behavior motivated by desire, action implies desire.

symphonology　A system of interpersonal ethics based on the terms and presuppositions of agreement. In any specific case, this will be the agreement that establishes the nature of the relationship between the parties involved in interaction.

system　The interrelationships of the elements that make up a whole.

term　A condition or stipulation that defines the nature and limits of an agreement" (American Heritage Dictionary, 1997).

triage　A triage situation is a situation calling for choices to be made when the benefits that can be brought about in the situation are limited. The choices may be choices among benefits or beneficiaries or both.

truth　The relationship of correspondence between an idea and the object of the idea.

uncertainty　The mental context of a dilemma. The right/best course of action may be action A or action B. But the superiority of one over the other is not clearly evident to the person who has to make the choice.

utilitarianism　"The theory that one should act as to promote the greatest happiness (pleasure) of the greatest number of people" (Angeles, 1992).

value　The object of an action that is motivated by an autonomous desire; that which is instrumental in the realization of a purpose.

violate　To violate a standard is to ignore or act against the character-structure that is signified by the standard. More generally, whenever one ignores or acts against that which is appropriate to an agreement, one violates the agreement.

virtue　A human excellence. "Action according to the nature of that which acts" (Spinoza, 1949). For instance, it is a virtue in a horse to run swiftly; it is a virtue in a boat not to sink; it is a virtue in a person to live rightly and well.

According to a purposive ethic, "virtue" refers to a person's ability to act to fulfill his or her rational desires.

vital Essentially related to the preservation or enhancement of life, as, for instance, a vital need or a vital desire.

volition The power to take uncompelled and purposeful actions.

whim A decision made on the analysis of subjective factors. A decision motivated by one's feelings or attitudes apart from the context.

REFERENCES

American heritage dictionary (3rd ed.). (1997). Boston: Houghton Mifflin.

Angeles, P. (1992). *Dictionary of philosophy*. New York: Harper Collins.

Pines, A., & Maslach, C. (1978). Characteristics of staff burn-out in mental health setting. *Hospital Community Psychiatry, 29,* 233–237.

McKeon, R. (Ed.). (1941). *The basic works of Aristotle*. New York: Random House.

Runes, D. D. (Ed.). (1983). *Dictionary of philosophy*. New York: Philosophical Library.

Siegel, B. (1993). Going native. *Hastings Center Report, 22*(1), 46.

Spinoza. (1949). *Ethics*. (J. Gutmann, Ed.). New York: Hafner Publishing. (Original work published 1675)

Index

Springer Publishing Company

Ethics in Community-Based Elder Care

Martha B. Holstein, PhD and **Phyllis Mitzen,** ACSW, LCSW, Editors

Caring for older people outside of institutions is the fastest growing sector of the US health care industry. Building upon their research study at the Park Ridge Center, in this volume editors Holstein and Mitzen along with a team of expert authors examine the complexities involved in developing an ethics for community-based long-term care and challenge policymakers to make it a more viable option for older people in need of care.

2001   304pp   0-8261-2297-3   *hardcover*
www.springerpub.com

536 Broadway, New York, NY 10012-3955 • (212) 431-4370 • Fax (212) 941-7842

Springer Publishing Company

End-of-Life Ethics and the Nursing Assistant

Eileen R. Chichin, PhD, RN, **Orah R. Burack,** MA
Ellen Olson, MD, and **Antonios Likourezos,** MA, MPH

This book describes a research-based project that was developed to assess Certified Nursing Assistants (CNAs) knowledge and attitudes about ethical issues and end-of-life decision-making and to provide educational intervention and support. CNAs provide most of the hands-on care in long-term facilities and, often over years, develop close relationships with residents. As a result, treatment termination and/or death can have a marked impact on CNAs.

Based on the project's findings, a workbook was designed to enable nursing homes to conduct an ethics education program for their CNAs. The workbook (contained in this book), Teaching End-Of-Life Ethics to CNAs, authored by Orah R. Burack and colleagues, has useful appendices including a questionnaire, ethics education instruction booklet with responses from the original study, an evaluation form, and a CNA ethics booklet.

Contents:
Foreword, by M. Mezey
• The Certified Nursing Assistant
• Respect for Autonomy
• Comfort Care
• Study Methods
• Study Results
• CNAs: How they see Themselves: How We See Them
• Respect for Autonomy: Opinions of Certified Nursing Assistants
• Comfort Care and the Certified Nursing Assistant
• CNAs' Evaluations of the Educational Ethics Program
• The Certified Nursing Assistant Support Group Program
• Implications of the Project: Where do We Go from Here
• Appendix

2000   224pp   0-8261-1307-9   hardcover
www.springerpub.com

536 Broadway, New York, NY 10012-3955 • (212) 431-4370 • Fax (212) 941-7842

Springer Publishing Company

Geriatrics and the Law, Third Edition
Understanding Patient Rights and Professional Responsibilities
Marshall B. Kapp, JD, MPH

"This updated Third Edition of Geriatrics and the Law by the leading scholar in Law and Old Age belongs on the desk of every hospital and long term care administrator, director of nursing, and medical director. It is the most comprehensive volume available on the topic. The book provides clearly written legal and ethical principles and their implications and applications."

—Elias S. Cohen
Executive Director, Community Service Systems, Inc.

Significant changes in the law are affecting patients' rights and professionals' responsibilities in providing clinical services to the elderly. This edition of Kapp's successful text continues to inform and sensitize health care professionals about the legal issues, and offers practical advice and guidance to practioners in a variety of disciplines.

The text has been thoroughly updated and, where appropriate, expanded. Topics woven into each chapter include: implications of the relevant statutes, regulations, judicial opinions, private guidelines, and discussion of new laws.

This practical book is a valuable and useful resource for practitioners, health care students, and educators. It contains extensive references and a helpful Appendix of Resources.

Contents: Demography and Epidemiology of Aging • Introduction to Law and the Legal System • Informed Consent and Truth Telling • Medical Record Keeping: Documentation, Patient Access, and Confidentiality • Financing Health Care for Older Persons • Disability Programs and Protections for Older Persons • Elder Abuse and Neglect • Involuntary Commitment, Guardianship, Protective Services, Representative Payees, and Power of Attorney • Medicolegal Problems in Caring for Nursing Home Residents • Legal Considerations in Home Health Care • Medicolegal Issues at the End of Life • Research with Older Human Subjects • Legal Services to Older Persons: Physician / Attorney Cooperation

1999   328pp.   0-8261-4532-9   hardcover
www.springerpub.com

536 Broadway, New York, NY 10012-3955 • (212) 431-4370 • Fax (212) 941-7842

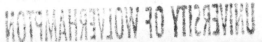

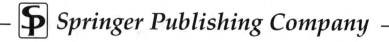

SP *Springer Publishing Company*

Ethics, Law, and Aging Review, Vol. 7

Liability Issues and Risk Management in Caring for Older Persons

Marshall B. Kapp, JD, MPH, Editor

Regulation and litigation regarding the health care of older persons is extensive and growing. This book comprehensively surveys and evaluates the various areas of the law and provides valuable guidance for managing legal risks while enhancing the quality of care delivered to older persons in the full range of clinical settings—nursing homes, assisted living, and ambulatory care.

Contents:

2001 216pp (est.) 0-8261-1457-1 hardcover
www.springerpub.com

536 Broadway, New York, NY 10012-3955 • (212) 431-4370 • Fax (212) 941-7842

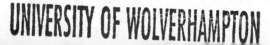